Surgery 2

For Churchill Livingstone

Publisher: Laurence Hunter
Project Editor: Barbara Simmons
Copy Editor: Jane Ward
Project Controller: Nancy Arnott
Design Direction: Erik Bigland, Charles Simpson
Indexer: Anne McCarthy
Page Layout: Gerard Heyburn

Churchill's Mastery of Medicine

Surgery 2

Edited by

John A. Dent

MMedEd MD FRCS (Ed)
Senior Orthopaedic Lecturer,
University of Dundee,
Dundee

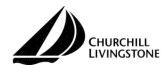

NEW YORK, EDINBURGH, LONDON, MADRID, MELBOURNE,
SAN FRANCISCO AND TOKYO 1997

CHURCHILL LIVINGSTONE
Medical Division of Pearson Professional Limited

Distributed in the United States of America by Churchill
Livingstone Inc., 650 Avenue of the Americas, New York, N.Y.
10011, and by associated companies, branches and
representatives throughout the world.

First published 1997

ISBN 0 443 05171 2

British Library of Cataloguing in Publication Data
A catalogue record for this book is available from the British
Library.

Library of Congress Cataloging in Publication Data
A catalog record for this book is available from the Library of
Congress.

Medical knowledge is constantly changing. As new information
becomes available, changes in treatment, procedures, equipment
and the use of drugs become necessary. The author and publisher
have, as far as it is possible, taken care to ensure that the
information given in this text is accurate and up to date.
However, readers are strongly advised to confirm that the
information, especially with regard to drug usage, complies with
current legislation and standards of practice.

The
publisher's
policy is to use
**paper manufactured
from sustainable forests**

Produced by Longman Singapore Publishers Pte Ltd
Printed in Singapore

Contributors

Robin L. Blair FRCS (Ed) FRCS (C) FACS
Consultant Otolaryngologist, University of Dundee,
Dundee

John A. Dent MMed Ed MD FRCS (Ed)
Senior Orthopaedic Lecturer, University of Dundee,
Dundee

Ivan Hanna MB ChB FRCS (Ed) FRCOphth
Consultant Ophthalmologist, Ayr Hospital, Ayr

Caroline J. MacEwen MB ChB MD FRCS FRCOphth
Consultant Ophthalmologist, Ninewells Hospital and
Medical School; Honorary Senior Lecturer, University
of Dundee, Dundee

Contents

Using this book

'What do I need to know about the surgical specialties?'
'Do I know the right things?'
'Can I remember the key points in the management of ...?'

These are the sort of questions which haunt us as exams approach but by then unfortunately there is seldom time to go back to extensive textbooks or sketchy lecture notes for the answers.

This is just the time when this new revision textbook comes in useful. In it you will find the 'core' information you require presented in a concise and systematic fashion which highlights the key facts you should know about any topic in a way which will help you remember them. But rather than simply giving you lots of facts to memorise, the principles of diagnosis and management are explained so that it becomes easier for you to work out the answers for yourself. The book does not aim to offer a complete 'syllabus'. It is impossible to draw boundaries around medical knowledge and learning as this is really a continuous process carried out throughout your medical career. With this in mind, you should aim to develop the ability to discern knowledge which you *need to know* from that which it is *nice to know*.

The aims of this introductory chapter are:

- to help plan your learning
- to show you how to use this book to increase your understanding as well as knowledge
- to realise how self-assessment can make learning easier and more enjoyable.

Layout and contents

The main part of the text describes topics considered to be of 'core' importance to the major subject areas. Within each chapter, essential information is presented in a set order with explanations and logical 'links' between topics. Where relevant, key facts about basic sciences, aetiology and pathological features are outlined. Where it is possible the clinical features are described under the key headings of 'Listen', 'Look', 'Feel' and 'Move'. Differential diagnosis and an approach to investigation are then described. Finally, the principles of management and the prognosis are presented. It is recognised that at the level of an undergraduate or newly qualified doctor a detailed understanding is not required; instead the ability to set out principles is all that is expected.

You will need to be sure that you are reaching the required standards, so in the final section of each chapter there are opportunities for you to check your knowledge and understanding. This self-assessment is in the form of multiple choice questions, patient management problems, case histories, data interpretation, picture quizzes and viva questions. All of these are centred around common clinical problems which are important in judging your performance as a doctor. Detailed answers are given. These answers will also contain some information and explanations that you will not find elsewhere, so you must do the assessment to get the most out of this book!

Using this book

If you are using this book as part of your exam preparations I suggest that your first task should be to map out on a sheet of paper three lists dividing the major subjects (corresponding to the chapter headings) into your strong, reasonable and weak areas. This will give you a rough outline of your revision schedule, which you must then fit in with the time available. Clearly, if your exams are looming large you will have to be ruthless in the time allocated to your strong areas. The major subjects should be further classified into individual topics. Encouragement to store information and to test your ongoing improvement is by the use of the self-assessment sections — you must not just read passively. It is important to keep checking your current level of knowledge, both strengths and weaknesses. This should be assessed objectively — self-rating in the absence of testing can be misleading. You may consider yourself strong in a particular area whereas it is more a reflection on how much you enjoy and are stimulated by the subject. Conversely you may be stronger in a subject than you would expect simply because the topic does not appeal to you.

It is a good idea to discuss topics and problems with colleagues/friends; the areas which you understand least well will soon become apparent when you try to explain them to someone else.

Approaching the examinations

The discipline of learning is closely linked to preparation for examinations. Many of us opt for a process of superficial learning that is directed towards retention of facts and recall under exam conditions because full understanding is often not required. It is much better if you try to acquire a deeper knowledge and understanding, combining the necessity of passing exams with longer term needs.

First, you need to know how you will be examined. Does the examination involve clinical assessment such as history taking and clinical examination? If you are sitting a written examination what are the length and types of question? How many must you answer and how much choice you will have?

Now you have to choose what sources you are going to use for your learning and revision. Textbooks come in different forms. At one extreme, there is the large reference book. This type of book should be avoided at this stage of revision and only used (if at all) for reference, when answers to questions cannot be found in smaller books. At the other end of the spectrum is the condensed 'lecture note' format, which often relies heavily on lists. Facts of this nature on their own are difficult to remember if they are not supported by understanding. In the middle of the range are the medium-sized textbooks. These are often of the most use whether you are approaching final University examinations or the first part of professional examinations. My advice is to choose one of the several medium-sized books on offer on the basis of which you find the most readable. The best approach is to combine your lecture notes, textbooks (appropriate to the level of study) and past examination papers as a framework for your preparation.

Armed with information about the format of the exams, a rough syllabus, your own lecture notes and some books that you feel comfortable in using, your next step is to map out the time available for preparation. You must be realistic, allow time for breaks and work *steadily*, not cramming. If you do attempt to cram, you have to realise that only a certain amount of information can be retained in your short-term memory, so as the classification of one condition moves in, the treatment of another moves out! Cramming simply retains facts. If the examination requires understanding you will be in trouble.

It is often a good idea to begin by outlining the topics to be covered and then attempt to summarise your knowledge about each in note form. In this way your existing knowledge will be activated and any gaps will become apparent. Self-assessment also helps determine the time to be allocated to each subject for exam preparation. If you are consistently scoring excellent marks in a particular subject it is not cost effective to spend a lot of time trying to achieve the 'perfect' mark.

In an essay it is many times easier to obtain the first mark (try writing your name) than the last. You should also try to decide on the amount of time assigned to each subject based on the likelihood of it appearing in the exam! Commonest things are usually commonest!

The main types of examination

Multiple choice questions

Unless very sophisticated, multiple choice questions test your recall of information. The aim is to gain the maximum marks from the knowledge that you can remember. The stem statement must be read with great care highlighting the 'little' words such as *only, rarely, usually, never* and *always*. Overlooking negatives, such as *not, unusual* and *unsuccessful* often cause marks to be lost. *May occur* has an entirely different connotation to *characteristic*. The latter may mean a feature which should be there and the absence of which would make you question the correctness of the diagnosis.

Remember to check the marking method before starting. Most multiple choice papers employ a negative system in which marks are lost for incorrect answers. The temptation is to adopt a cautious approach answering a relatively small number of questions. However, this can lead to problems as we all make simple mistakes or even disagree vehemently with the answer in the computer! Caution may lead you to answer too few questions to obtain a pass after the marks have been deducted for incorrect answers.

Short notes

Short notes are not negatively marked. Predetermined marks are given for each important key fact. Nothing is gained for style or superfluous information. The aim is to set out your knowledge in an ordered *concise* manner. Do not devote too much time to a single question thereby neglecting the rest, and remember to limit your answer to the question that has been set.

Essays

Similar comments apply to essays, but marks may be awarded for logical development of an argument or theme. Conversely, good marks will not be obtained for an essay that is a set of unconnected statements. Always plan your essay answer. Length matters little if there is no cohesion. It is even more important in an examination based on essays to manage your time carefully. *All questions must be given equal weight.* A brilliant answer in one essay will not compensate for not attempting another because time runs out.

Data interpretation

Data interpretation involves the application of knowledge to solve a problem. In your revision you should aim for an understanding of principles; it is impossible to memorise all the different data combinations. In an exam, a helpful approach is to translate numbers into a description; for example a serum potassium of 2.8 mmol/l is *low* and the ECG tracing of a heart rate of 120/min shows a *tachy*cardia. This type of question is usually not negatively marked so put down an answer even if you are far from sure that it is right.

Slide picture questions

Pattern recognition is the first step in a picture quiz. This should be coupled with a systematic approach looking for, and listing, abnormalities. For example the general appearance of the skeleton as well as the local appearance of the individual bones and any soft tissue shadows can be examined in any X-ray. Make an attempt to describe what you see even if you are in doubt. Use any additional statements or data which accompany the X-rays as they give a clue to the answer required.

Patient management problems

A more sophisticated form of exam question is an evolving case of history with information being presented sequentially and you being asked to give a response at each stage. They are constructed so that a wrong response in the first part of the questions does not mean that no more marks can be obtained from the subsequent parts. Each part should stand on its own. Patient management problems are designed to test the recall and application of knowledge through an understanding of the principles involved.

Vivas

Examples of viva questions are given together with notes on their answers. The viva examination can be a nerve-wracking experience. You are normally faced with two examiners who may react with irritation, boredom or indifference to what you say. You may feel that the viva has gone well and yet you fail, or more commonly, you think that the exam has gone terribly because of the apparent attitude of the examiners.

Your main aim during the viva should be to control the examiners' questioning so they constantly ask you about things you know. Despite what is often said, you can prepare for this form of exam. Questions are liable to take one of a small number of forms centred around subjects that cannot be examined in a traditional clinical exam.

During the viva there are certain techniques which help in making a favourable impression. When discussing patient management, it is better to say 'I would do this' rather than 'the book says this'. You should try and strike a balance between saying too little and too much. It is important to try not to go off the topic. Aim to keep your answers short and to the point. It is worthwhile pausing for a few seconds to collect your thoughts before launching into an answer. Do not be afraid to say 'I don't know'; most examiners will want to change tack to see what you do know about.

Conclusions

You should amend your framework for using this book according to your own needs and the examinations you are facing. Whatever approach you adopt, your aim should be for an understanding of the principles involved rather than rote learning of a large number of poorly connected facts.

Orthopaedics

Section

1

Musculoskeletal
trauma

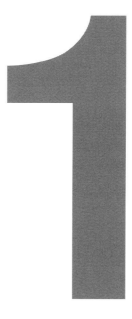

1.1 Clinical examination

The arrival of a patient with multiple injuries in the Accident and Emergency department is not infrequently accompanied by much ill-coordinated activity on the part of the receiving staff.

This type of action is not necessarily in the best interests of the patient and tends to delay rapid assessment and initiation of life-saving measures. A uniform coordinated approach is advocated by the Advanced Trauma Life Support (ATLS) System, whose routine method of efficiently managing such patients should become second nature to the medical and nursing staff who may be called upon to attend the patient with musculoskeletal trauma.

After initial assessment of injuries and appropriate resuscitation, the importance of a 'second-look' examination should be emphasised because it is at this stage that additional incidental injuries will be discovered.

On all occasions of patient interaction, the clinical skills of 'listen', 'look', 'feel' and 'move' should be followed.

Emergency treatment

The first few hours after injury is the time in which life can be saved if emergency measures are effectively applied. This emergency treatment of the multiply injured patient is best executed if the members of the resuscitation team follow the principles promoted by the ATLS system:

- airway and cervical spine control
- breathing
- circulation.

Followed by:

- disorder (neurological disorder)

- exposure/environmental control.

Airway and cervical spine control
The airway should be cleared of any obstructions such as dentures or vomit and in the comatose patient the tongue should be prevented from blocking the pharynx by holding the jaw forwards. An oropharyngeal or nasopharyngeal tube is often necessary but endotracheal intubation, cricothyroidotomy (Fig. 1) or a tracheostomy may be required if the upper airway is obstructed. The cervical cord must be protected by sand bags or by manually steadying the neck before it can be safely immobilised in a rigid cervical collar.

Breathing
Observe chest expansion, spontaneous ventilation and any abnormal movements of the chest wall, such as paradoxical movement, flail segment or a penetrating wound.

Circulation
Bleeding should be controlled by pressure dressings and elevation. Improvised tourniquets are too dangerous. A fast-flowing intravenous infusion should be instituted in a large peripheral vein; if necessary, a cutdown on a peripheral vein is required. A volume challenge with an intravenous crystalloid is the initial treatment of hypotension. Later cross-matched blood may be required. Passing a urinary catheter allows accurate monitoring of fluid balance and relieves the agitation caused by bladder distension.

Disorder (neurological disorder)
A rapid but thorough examination for evidence of head injury is carried out. The Glasgow Coma Scale is commonly used. This records the patient's motor, verbal and eye movement responses to stimulation. Evidence of spinal cord or peripheral nerve injury can be sought at this stage.

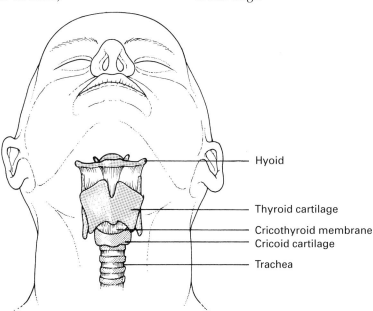

Hyoid

Thyroid cartilage

Cricothyroid membrane
Cricoid cartilage

Trachea

Fig. 1
A cricothyroidotomy can be made through the cricothyroid membrane between the cricoid and thyroid cartilages.

Exposure/environmental control
The entire patient must be exposed for thorough examination to exclude the presence of any additional injuries. The extent and depth of burns can be charted at this stage. Do not forget to examine the perineum and the back. Once this is done, steps must be taken to keep the patient warm. Recording of vital signs should be commenced.

Radiographic examination
Radiographs of chest, pelvis and lateral cervical spine are always required. Radiographs of other regions can be delayed until resuscitation is completed.

Open fractures

Open fractures require urgent treatment if bacterial invasion of the wound is to be avoided. Open fractures are classified according to their degree of contamination and soft tissue damage.

Management
Management can be divided into several steps:

- wound excision
  — irrigation: high pressure irrigation of the wound with saline is the initial step
  — debridement: all devitalised tissue, especially muscle, is excised and any dirt is washed from the wound
  — antibiotics: intravenous prophylactic antibiotics are commenced

- reduction
  — the bony fragments are aligned into normal position

- stabilisation
  — stabilisation of a fracture may be achieved by external or internal techniques. Once the wound has been cleaned surgically and the fracture reduced an appropriate method of fixation must be selected. If a radical debridement has been carried out many orthopaedic surgeons would select rigid

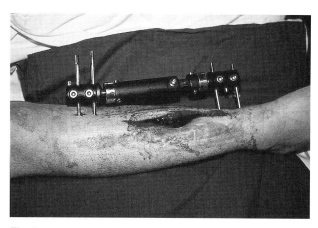

Fig. 2
External fixator used to stabilise an open tibial fracture without hindering access to the wound.

internal fixation of the fracture and primary skin cover using a local or a free flap as necessary. An external fixator (Fig. 2) is useful if the wound is to be left open or a 'second look' operation to excise more dead tissue is anticipated in 24 hours' time.

Complications
Complications can be divided into categories (see p. 15). Those particularly associated with open fractures include:

- wound infection
- chronic osteitis
- non union.

Compartment syndrome

Bleeding from a comminuted closed fracture of a long bone may increase the pressure in the adjacent fascial compartment. In the leg, there are four compartments (Fig. 3) and in the forearm two compartments. Bleeding from the bone and swelling of damaged muscle within these compartments increase pressure on the artery and nerve passing through them and result in progressive muscle and nerve ischaemia.

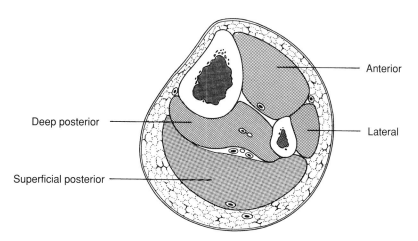

Anterior

Deep posterior

Lateral

Superficial posterior

Fig. 3
Deep fascial compartments in the leg.

Clinical features

- Listen—pain more severe than would be expected from the injury alone
- Look—tense swollen limb
- Feel—altered sensation and diminished pulses distally will eventually be present
- Move—resisted passive stretching of the muscle bellies in the compartment involved.

Diagnosis

A pressure transducer can be introduced to monitor pressure within the compartment but the clinical features remain the most important in making the diagnosis.

Management

If the removal of circumferential dressings is ineffective, an urgent fasciotomy is required to relieve the raised compartment pressure. In the lower leg, this can be achieved by a partial fibulectomy. In the forearm, the flexor and extensor compartments must be decompressed separately. The skin wound can be left open to be closed or covered with a split thickness skin graft a few days later when the swelling has subsided.

Complications

- Volkmann's ischaemic contracture
- persisting nerve damage.

Second-look examination

After initial emergency assessment, it is important to carry out a second-look examination to identify any additional injuries.

1.2 Fracture types

The most important observation to make about a fracture is whether it is open or closed. In closed fractures, the skin is intact but in open fractures there are varying degrees of severity of contamination and soft tissue damage (see above). It is easy to think of the bone injury in isolation, especially when looking at a radiograph, but it must be remembered that the soft tissues have also been damaged by the injuring force. An accurate history will tell something about the mechanism of the injury and about the amount of energy imparted to the bone and soft tissues by the injuring force. The radiograph will show the pattern of the resulting fracture. Both the history and the radiograph will help in making a decision on the probable stability of the fracture and the extent of damage to be expected in the surrounding soft tissues.

Mechanism of injury

Direct violence

When direct violence is applied to a bone, the overlying skin and soft tissues are likely to be broken and damaged.

A small force to a localised area, such as from a blow with a stick to the forearm, will bruise or break the overlying skin and cause a transverse fracture usually of the ulna (Fig. 4).

A large force to a large area, such as from being hit by a car bumper, will produce a comminuted fracture with extensive soft tissue damage, crushing and devitalisation. A large force to a small area from a missile injury will produce severe damage to bone and soft tissues in a localised area.

Indirect violence

The injuring force is applied to the limb at a distance from where the fracture occurs. Examples are a twisting injury to the tibia (Fig. 5), often caused when the foot is

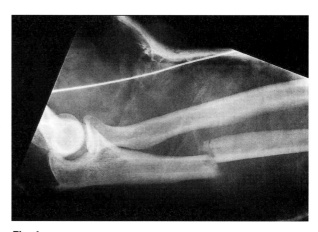

Fig. 4
Transverse fracture of the middle third of the ulna following a direct blow on the forearm.

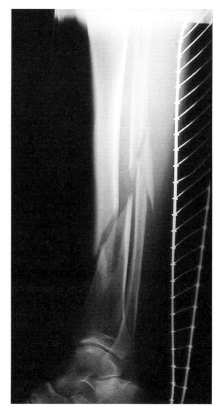

Fig. 5
Spiral fracture of the tibia and fibula.

jammed (for instance in a football tackle) while the body twists and falls to the side. The fracture is less likely to be open than one caused by direct violence. The soft tissue envelope, however, can be extensively stripped from the bone.

When angulatory forces are directed to the limb, a transverse fracture results which may have intact periosteum on the compression side but a tear in the periosteal sleeve on the distraction side.

Other mechanisms of injury include stress fractures from repetitive forces being applied to the bone, as seen in the 'march fracture' of the second metatarsal.

Fracture patterns

Transverse fractures. These arise when angulatory forces are applied to the limb, for instance by levering it over a fulcrum (e.g. the leg caught between the rungs when falling from a stepladder) or a fall on the out-stretched hand. Direct blows to an isolated area of the bone can also cause a transverse fracture.

Spiral fractures. Twisting forces create spiral fractures (e.g. the foot blocked in a football tackle while the player falls to the side).

Comminuted fractures. These are high-energy fractures and are inherently unstable (e.g. the leg hit by a car bumper).

Crush fractures. These occur as a result of longitudinal (axial) forces and are seen in areas of cancellous bone, such as the tibial condyles and vertebrae (e.g. a patient who falls from a height and lands on the feet may fracture the os calcis and vertebrae) (Fig. 6).

Oblique fractures. These are caused by a combination of twisting, angulation and compression forces.

Greenstick fractures. These transverse fractures occur in children as a result of angulatory forces (Fig. 7). One cortex is broken but the cortex on the compression side is merely buckled.

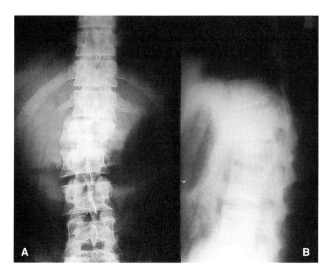

Fig. 6
A. Crush fracture of the body of the first lumbar vertebra.
B. View of the same injury showing the displacement associated with the crush fracture.

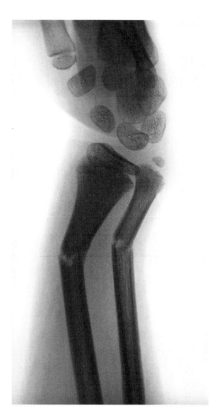

Fig. 7
Greenstick fractures of the radius and ulna in a child.

Malalignment

A fracture may be:

- displaced
- angulated
- shortened
- rotated.

Displacement. In a displaced fracture, the distal fragment is displaced in a sagittal or coronal plane relative to the proximal fragment but without any angulation (Fig. 8). The overall alignment of the limb is satisfactory. If the fracture is stable then healing will proceed without residual deformity as the fracture remodels.

Angulation. The distal fragment may be angulated forwards or backwards, laterally or medially (Fig. 9). Only a few degrees of lateral or medial (valgus or varus) angulation are acceptable. No remodelling will take place in this plane but it will if the angulation is in an antero-posterior plane.

Shortening. In a completely displaced fracture, the bone fragments will override each other and the limb will shorten (Fig. 10). Shortening also occurs in comminuted fractures where there is impaction of the articular surface into the metaphysis.

Rotation. The distal fragment of a fracture may be rotated on the proximal fragment. A radiograph showing the full length of the injured limb will make it easier to recognise this deformity (Fig. 11).

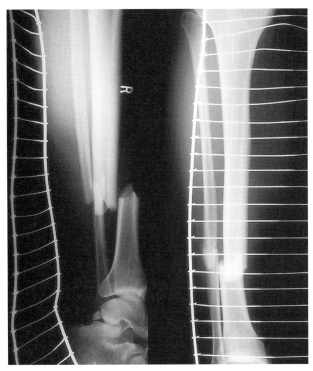

Fig. 8
Transverse fractures of the distal tibia and fibula with 100%
displacement but with no angulatory deformity.

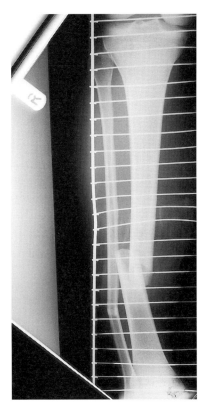

Fig. 9
Transverse fracture of the distal tibia and fibula with marked
varus angulation at the fracture site.

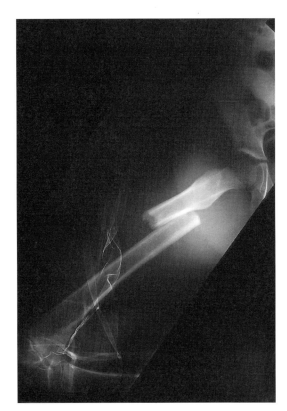

Fig. 10
Transverse fracture of the upper third of the femur in a child with
considerable shortening at the fracture site due to overriding of
the bone ends.

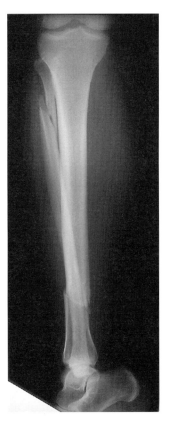

Fig. 11
Rotary deformity of a fracture of the distal tibia and proximal
fibula. The radiograph shows an antero-posterior view of the
knee with a lateral view of the ankle!

1.3 Methods of treatment

Fracture stabilisation may be achieved by external or internal techniques:

External

- traction
- splint (plaster cast)
- functional brace
- external fixator.

Internal

- intermedullary rod
- plates
- screws
- wires.

Traction

Traction is used to overcome muscle spasm and so allow the bone fragments to realign in the soft tissue envelope.

Skin traction to a maximum of 5 kg can be applied to the leg by fastening the weights to adhesive strapping around the limb. This is used only as a temporary measure in adults but is used for definitive treatment of femoral fractures in young children.

In skeletal traction, weights are applied to the limb via a pin passed through the tibial tuberosity for traction on the femur or through the os calcis for traction on the tibia. The patient's limb can be nursed in a Thomas splint and the traction cords tied to its end. This is fixed traction. Alternatively, the patient can lie free in bed with the fracture supported in a cradle while traction applied distally is provided by weights which hang to the floor round a pulley at the foot of the bed. This is balanced traction (Fig. 12).

Advantages

- simple to erect
- safe to use.

Disadvantages

- prolonged immobilisation with associated problems of pressure sores, osteoporosis, muscle wasting and joint stiffness
- distraction of the fracture.

Plaster casts

Plaster of Paris immobilisation is the most common type of splintage to hold a fracture after it has been manipulated into a satisfactory position. Three-point fixation is required to prevent subsequent loss of the position achieved.

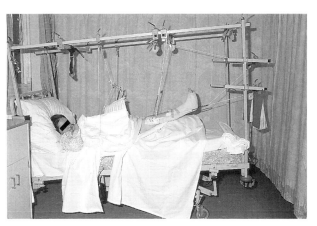

Fig. 12
Balanced traction. The femoral fracture is nursed in the canvas cradle while traction is applied distally via the tibial tuberosity.

Advantages

- easy to use
- cheap
- readily available.

Disadvantages

- rigid fixation is not possible so the bone fragments can slip
- pressure sores beneath the plaster
- stiff joints
- peripheral swelling.

Functional brace

A close-fitting plaster cuff that maintains the girth of the limb will prevent shortening at the fracture site (Fig. 13). By preventing the limb from widening, the length of the limb and hence the position of the fracture are maintained. For some fractures, hinges are accurately placed at the elbow or knee joints to allow motion at the joint while the fracture heals.

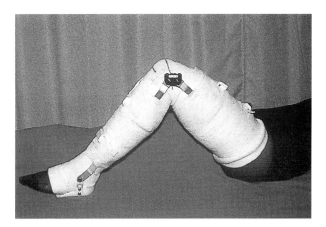

Fig. 13
Femoral fracture controlled by a functional brace. The hinges at the knee and ankle allow early rehabilitation of the joints.

Advantages

- allows joint movement
- prevents muscle stiffness and wasting.

Disadvantages

- accurate fitting is required.

External fixation

Threaded pins are drilled into the bone on either side of the fracture and fixed via universal joints to a rigid bar near the skin surface.

Advantages

- quick and easy to apply
- allows access to wounds and observation of the skin surface.

Disadvantages

- pin tracking infection
- increased risk of infection if intermedullary fixation is subsequently used
- delayed union if the fixation is too rigid.

Internal fixation

Internal fixation can be achieved by various mechanisms:

- screws
- plates
- intermedullary rods
- wire.

Screws. Lag screws are used to secure fragments of bone together, such as avulsion fractures of the medial malleolus.

Plates. A direct compression plate (DCP) is used to secure long bone fractures, such as forearm fractures. The direct compression design produces compression at the fracture site, which stimulates osteosynthesis (Fig. 14).

Intermedullary nail. These are used for tibial and femoral fractures. The cortex is reamed under radiographic control. The nail is locked into the bone by transverse bolts above and below the fracture, which controls the rotation and length of the bone.

Wire. Tension band wire is used to secure avulsion fractures of the patella and olecranon.

Advantages

- anatomical reduction
- early active mobilisation.

Disadvantages

- infection
- wound breakdown
- non-union
- delayed union
- considerable expertise is required for successful use of these techniques

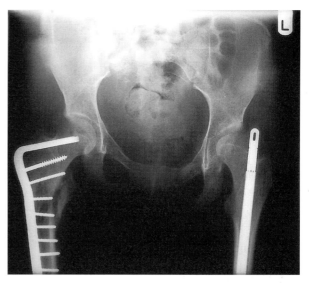

Fig. 14
Complex bilateral fractures of the femoral treated by an angled blade plate on the right and on the left by an intramedullary rod.

- the fixation device produces a stress riser which may lead to subsequent fractures
- osteoporosis
- cutting out.

Internal fixation gives the best chance of early rehabilitation and return to normal life, and is especially useful for problem patients and problem fractures. Problem patients include those with:

- multiple injuries
- prolonged unconsciousness.

Problem fractures include:

- intra-articular fractures
- unstable fractures
- pathological fractures.

1.4 Long bone fractures

Clinical features

The characteristic features of a fracture of any long bone are:

- Listen — a history of trauma
    — pain
    — bruising
- Look — deformity
    — swelling
- Feel — diminished pulses and altered sensation may be present
- Move — loss of function
    — crepitus.

In addition, there may be local bruising, and examination of the periphery may show diminished pulses and areas of altered sensation.

The most important fact to establish is whether the fracture is open or closed. The presence of a skin wound which communicates with the fracture means that the fracture is an open one and risks of infection are increased. In grade one open fractures, the skin is merely punctured but the wound is clean and the skin and soft tissues are not crushed. In grade two open fractures, the wound is larger, grossly contaminated and there is more soft tissue damage. In grade three open fractures, there is extensive periosteal stripping, muscle crushing and contamination. Grade three open fractures have been further classified into different degrees of severity.

Diagnosis

Diagnosis is usually made clinically but radiological examination is required to confirm the configuration of the fracture and plan future treatment.

Management

Non-operative management

- plaster cast
- traction
- functional brace.

Operative management

- internal fixation
- external fixation, see page 40.

Complications

Complications can be considered as the following categories:

- early
- late
- local
  systemic — adult respiratory distress syndrome, fat embolus, pulmonary embolus.
- bony — chronic osteitis, non-union, delayed union, malunion
- soft tissue — wound breakdown and infection, heterotopic calcification, compartment syndrome.

1.5 Spinal injuries

Spinal injuries usually occur in falls from a height or in road traffic accidents. They must always be suspected if a patient has suffered multiple, high-energy injuries, especially if there has been a blow to the head.

Cervical spine

The bony injury to the cervical spine may be complicated by damage to the cervical cord.

Clinical features

- Listen — there may be a history of a fall from a height or other type of deceleration injury
- Look — abdominal respiration without thoracic expansion
- Feel — numbness to touch sensation in all dermatomes below the level of the injury
- Move — the patient is unable to move the arms or legs voluntarily.

Diagnosis

X-ray of the cervical spine shows the level of the injury which may be either a subluxation or a dislocation (Fig. 15). The extent of the bony injury can be further defined by CT scan and the soft tissue injury by MRI or CT myelography.

Management

Patients with cervical cord injury

Emergency treatment involves urethral catheterisation, intravenous infusion to maintain circulating volume and skull traction to affect reduction of the dislocated cervical spine. After several days, the permanent level of the quadriplegia becomes apparent. Expert nursing care is required to avoid bed sores, chest infection, urinary tract infection, constipation and demoralisation.

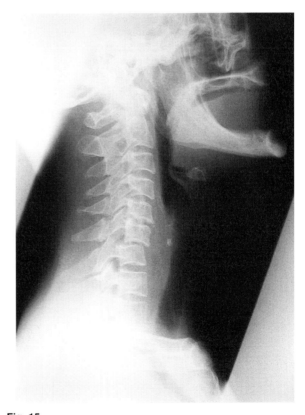

Fig. 15
Lateral X-ray of the cervical spine showing all the cervical vertebrae. There is a subluxation of C6 on C7.

Reconstructive surgery utilising functioning muscle groups can sometimes restore some function to the hand and elbow.

Complications

- renal calculi
- urinary tract infection
- pressure sores
- impotence.

Thoraco-lumbar spine

High-velocity injuries can cause fractures of the thoracic or lumbar spine without neurological damage, but in cases of fracture dislocation the spinal cord is often damaged, resulting in paraplegia.

Clinical features

- Listen — history of a fall or road traffic accident
- Look — there is swelling and bruising over the spine at the site of the injury
- Feel — local tenderness
- Move — loss of voluntary movement below the spinal level of the injury
  Bladder function is impaired causing urinary retention.

Diagnosis

Radiological examination confirms the level of the spinal injury and shows the configuration of the fracture. As before, computerised tomography (CT), and MRI will show the extent of cord and nerve root compression by the bony fragments.

Management

Particular care is required to prevent further damage to the cord and to avoid bed sores. Urethral catheterisation is required. The permanent level of the neurological deficit becomes apparent over a short period of time. Surgical stabilisation of the bony injury may be appropriate for local pain relief, but it does not reverse the neurological damage.

Patients will require a wheelchair for mobility, but with enthusiastic support a great deal of independence can be enjoyed.

Complications
- renal calculi
- urinary tract infection
- pressure sores
- impotence.

Self-assessment: questions

Multiple choice questions

1. Functional cast-bracing of a femoral shaft fracture:
   a. Should not be applied before 10 weeks after the injury
   b. Allows early knee flexion
   c. Allows weight bearing
   d. Should be ischial-bearing
   e. Has the recognised complication of inducing quadriceps wasting

2. In the conservative treatment of fractures:
   a. Joint stiffness is associated with plaster cast immobilisation only when this has been applied too tightly
   b. In a patient with a forearm fracture treated in plaster, pain on passive extension of the fingers is caused by impingement of flexor muscles at the fracture site
   c. Malalignment of 5° in a tibial fracture in any plane is acceptable
   d. Functional bracing is a recognised treatment of tibial shaft fractures after the first 3 to 4 weeks
   e. A recognised method of treatment of complex intra-articular fractures is traction and active mobilisation of the affected joint

3. Open fractures:
   a. Are often treated by delayed primary suture of the soft tissues
   b. Wound toilet should be performed within 6 hours
   c. Are associated with accelerated healing potential
   d. Should not be treated by internal fixation
   e. Are best treated by saucerisation of bone and soft tissues

Case histories

History 1

> A 20-year-old man has been thrown from his motorcycle in a collision with your car. He is lying on his back motionless at the roadside.

1. What is the first thing to do?
2. List what should be done next in order of priority
3. Describe the method by which he can be safely moved once the ambulance arrives

History 2

> A ward nurse calls you during the night about a patient complaining of pain beneath his plaster. He had a closed fracture of his tibia manipulated and put in an above knee plaster earlier in the day.

1. List the key points of a physical examination
2. What therapeutic measures should be instituted?

Picture question

The radiograph shows both tibiae of a patient (Fig. 16). How would you describe the configuration of the fractures? What associated complications can be expected?

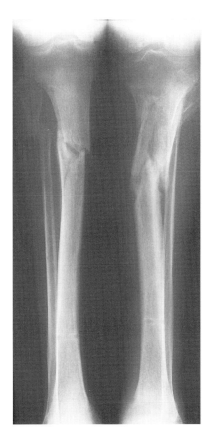

Fig. 16
This patient was hit on both shins by a car bumper.

Essay questions

1. Describe the features of a greenstick fracture, indicating how this injury differs from a transverse fracture in an adult.
2. List the advantages and disadvantages of internal fixation of fractures and illustrate your answer by reference to a bimalleolar fracture of the ankle.

Viva questions

1. How would you manage a grade two open fracture of the tibia?
2. How would you manage a transverse fracture of the femoral shaft in a 10-year-old child?
3. What are the main points of the early management of a patient with cervical spine injury?

Self-assessment: answers

Multiple choice answers

1. a. **False**. A favourable femoral shaft fracture which has been treated conservatively in traction for 4 to 6 weeks should then be suitable for application of a functional brace.
   b. **True**.
   c. **True**.
   d. **True**. This design allows load sharing between the orthosis and the fractured femur.
   e. **False**. Muscles are able to exercise in the functional brace so that wasting is avoided.

2. a. **False**. Joint stiffness is associated with immobility, not ischaemia from a tightly applied cast.
   b. **False**. The presence of pain on passive extension of the fingers suggests ischemia of the flexor muscle bellies and an impending compartment syndrome.
   c. **True**. This minor degree of malalignment is acceptable. More angulation is acceptable in the antero-posterior plane as remodelling can be expected, but greater degrees of varus or valgus malalignment will not remodel.
   d. **True**. The above knee plaster can be changed to a patella tendon-bearing cast, which is a type of functional brace, at 3 to 4 weeks after the injury.
   e. **True**. In cases where there are local or general contraindications to operation, then traction and active mobilisation will help realign complex intra-articular fractures and allow remoulding of the articular surfaces.

3. a. **True**. It is wise to leave the wound open for 24 hours so that a further inspection can be made to look for signs of infection or muscle ischaemia.
   b. **True**. After 6 hours, significant bacterial colonisation of the wound has taken place but before this time it can be prevented by debridement, irrigation and prophylactic antibiotics.
   c. **False**.
   d. **False**. Internal fixation is not contraindicated provided thorough wound debridement and irrigation are carried out and appropriate antibiotics prescribed prophylactically.
   e. **False**. This is the treatment for chronic osteitis.

Case history answers

History 1

1. When first attending a road accident, it is important to take measures to ensure the safety of yourself and the victim from other vehicles or from fire as a result of spilled petrol.

2. Your management of the patient in order of priority would then follow the ATLS system of airway, breathing and circulation, etc. The airway must be guarded by sweeping obstructions from the mouth. Measures should be taken in the unconscious patient to prevent the tongue falling backwards. Breathing should be observed and any penetrating wound in the chest covered with an occlusive dressing. Bleeding should be controlled by pressure dressings and elevation. If necessary, cardiopulmonary resuscitation should be commenced and, if available, a large-bore intravenous catheter should be introduced into a large peripheral vein for administration of intravenous fluids.

3. When it is necessary to move the patient, the cervical spine must be manually held steady at all times until a rigid surgical collar can be applied. A spinal board or other firm support is required to splint the patient's pelvis, spine and head while being moved.

History 2

1. From the history you suspect a development of a compartment syndrome in the leg. Your physical examination includes observing the toes for swelling and congestion. Passive dorsiflexion should be carried out to see if this produces pain in the calf. Sensation should be checked on the dorsum of the toes and the first web space.

2. If symptoms are not relieved by release of the plaster cast then a formal fasciotomy should be arranged. Although intracompartmental pressures can be measured these must not delay surgical decompression if this is indicated clinically.

Picture answer

The radiograph shows a comminuted fracture of the upper third of both tibiae. This fracture pattern in the presence of a closed injury may result in bleeding into the fascial compartments and the development of a compartment syndrome.

Essay answers

1. In a greenstick fracture, the cortex is fractured on the distraction side but buckled on the compression side of the bone. A similar angulating force in an adult would result in a transverse fracture extending completely across the bone. The compression side will fracture in an adult rather than undergo plastic deformation as it does in a child.

2. The advantages of internal fixation are anatomical reduction and the ability to carry out early active

mobilisation of the joint. The disadvantages include infection, wound breakdown, delayed union and implant failure. In a bimalleolar fracture of the ankle, the use of a neutralisation plate on the lateral malleolus and a lagged malleolar screw on the medial malleolus will restore the configuration of the ankle mortis and allow early active mobilisation of the joint, which will aid healing of the articular cartilage.

Viva answers

1. An open fracture of the tibia should be managed by wound irrigation, debridement and prophylactic antibiotics. High-pressure irrigation with copious volumes of saline is preferred. The wound edges should be excised and the wound cleaned. Any devitalised tissue should be excised. A prophylactic course of appropriate antibiotics should be instituted. In a more severe fracture, a second-look operation should be planned 24 hours later.

2. A transverse femoral shaft fracture in a 10-year-old child would best be managed by conservative treatment using traction. The limb is nursed on a Thomas splint using skin traction. This is usually sufficient to align the fragments while fracture healing occurs.

3. The initial management of a patient with a cervical spine injury involves instituting traction on the cervical spine by either a halter or by skull tongs. The patient's neck must be kept immobilised to prevent extending the damage to the spinal cord or nerve roots. General management of the patient includes restoration of circulating volume by intravenous infusion, urethral catheterisation and care of pressure points.

Fractures in the elderly

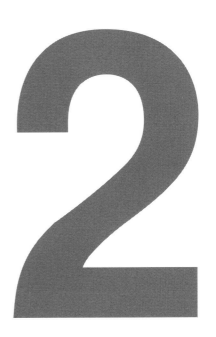

2.1 Clinical examination

The full clinical examination of an elderly patient is often difficult. History taking may be complicated by deafness, dementia or debility, so the physical examination must be sufficiently extensive to identify the presence of other medical or surgical conditions.

The physical examination of the injured part involves the usual sequence of 'look, feel and move' but in the presence of a suspected pathological fracture the local physical examination should be extended to include the neck, breasts, chest, abdomen and rectum.

Osteoporosis

Osteoporosis in the ageing skeleton is a primary cause of the increased frequency of fractures in the elderly.

Osteoporosis is not necessarily associated with age, but it is associated with a decreased level of mobility, which may be associated with older age groups. Lack of stress on the bones and dietary deficiency contribute to osteoporosis but the most important cause in elderly females is postmenopausal hormone change. Unsteadiness of the feet for whatever reason and syncopal attacks lead to an increased likelihood of the patient suffering a fracture from a simple fall at home.

2.2 Distal radius fractures

The Colles' fracture is the classical injury seen in the postmenopausal female, usually in the seventh decade of life. The fracture may be comminuted and may extend into the radio-carpal joint, the inferior radio-ulnar joint or both.

Clinical features

- Listen — there is usually a history of a fall on the outstretched hand
- Look — the distal fragment of the radius and the attached carpal bones are usually displaced posteriorly to create the characteristic 'dinner fork' deformity of the wrist (Fig. 17). There is often swelling and bruising. Radial deviation and supination of the distal fragment may also be present.
- Feel — tenderness
    - the median nerve may be compressed, producing altered sensation in the radial three and a half digits
- Move — the patient is reluctant to move the wrist
    - crepitus may be apparent.

Diagnosis

An antero-posterior and a true lateral radiograph of the wrist are required to confirm the diagnosis (Fig. 18A).

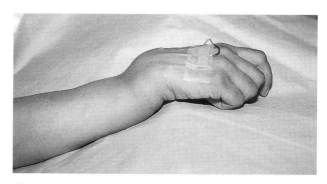

Fig. 17
Classical dinner fork deformity of a Colles' fracture.

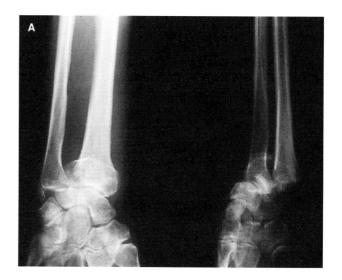

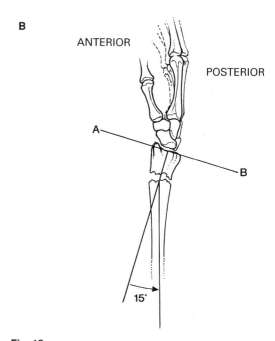

Fig. 18
A. Lateral and antero-posterior radiograph Colles' fracture, showing the posterior displacement of the distal radial fragment and shortening of the radius. **B**. Method of measuring the degree of angulation present at the fracture site.

There is often impaction at the fracture site as the distal fragment is displaced proximally. This produces shortening of the radius, and the ulna now appears relatively long.

Management

A casualty officer dealing with this injury needs to decide whether the fracture requires to be reduced. To do this the amount of displacement at the fracture site must be assessed to see if it is acceptable and can be simply splinted, or whether an anatomical position should be sought by means of manipulation under anaesthesia.

If the fracture is not manipulated or 'reduced', the fracture will still unite but in an abnormal position. Moderate degrees of displacement may be acceptable, but more severe malunion will cause limitation of wrist function, especially flexion and supination. Figure 18B shows the method of measuring the degree of angulation present at the fracture site between the two fragments. The line AB has been drawn across the articular surface of the radius on the lateral radiograph. A perpendicular line to this transects the line drawn along the long axis of the proximal fragment of the radius; usually 15° of angulation is acceptable. Angulation greater than this is usually corrected by manipulation.

Manipulation of the fracture requires reversal of the direction of the deforming force that produced the original injury. After manipulating a fracture into an acceptable position, there are several ways available to hold this position until the fracture has united.

Usually a Colles' fracture can be held in place with a plaster of Paris cast. This holds the wrist in the reduced position of flexion, ulnar deviation and pronation. This position is exactly the opposite from the displaced position of the Colles' fracture.

A minor degree of malunion is acceptable as the functional result may be unimpaired. In some cases, the fracture may be very unstable when manipulated and consequently difficult to hold in correct position in relation to the ulna by plaster of Paris alone. In such cases percutaneous pins or an external fixator may be used to splint the fracture until union is achieved. The external fixator can be applied to the second metacarpal and the proximal radius (Fig. 19).

Very rarely, open reduction and internal fixation of a Colles' fracture is required. A buttress plate on the radius and a bone graft may be necessary to hold this position.

After 4 to 6 weeks of immobilisation, the wrist is stiff and a period of physiotherapy is often required to regain a full range of mobilisation. The patient is required actively to attempt dorsiflexion, palmar flexion and supination/pronation exercises and also to exercise the elbow and shoulder.

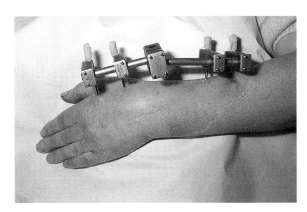

Fig. 19
Comminuted fracture of the distal radius in a younger patient stabilised by an external fixator which holds the radius at its correct length and position.

Complications

Complications can be divided into those occurring early and late:

- early complications
  — median nerve compression
- late complications
  — malunion
  — elbow and wrist stiffness
  — frozen shoulder
  — spontaneous rupture of extensor pollicis longus
  — reflex sympathetic dystrophy (Sudek's atrophy).

2.3 Upper humerus fractures

A history of a fall on the outstretched hand in a lady in her seventies is a common presentation of a fracture of the upper humerus.

Classification
- intracapsular fractures occur at the anatomical neck with avulsion of one or both tuberosities
- extracapsular fractures occur at the surgical neck, the narrowest portion of the proximal humerus.

The blood supply to the humeral head may be disrupted in intracapsular fractures because of its separation from the greater and lesser tuberosities and their soft tissue attachments and because of the fracture in the shaft below it. The head is liable to undergo avascular necrosis in the same way as that seen in subcapital fractures of the head of the femur (see p. 26).

Clinical features

There is bruising and swelling over the shoulder with loss of abduction because of pain. Axillary nerve damage may be present and must be searched for by elicit-

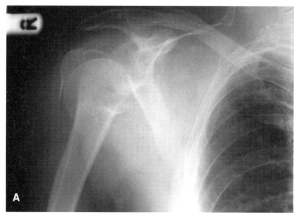

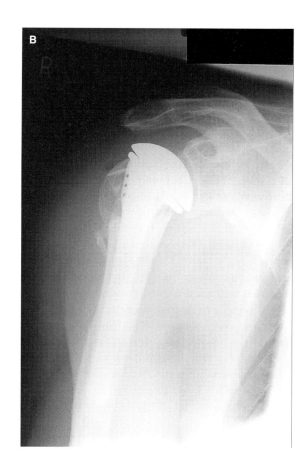

Fig. 20
A. Four-part fracture of the humerus in a 65-year-old man. The articular surface of the humerus is rotated away from the glenoid.
B. Fracture seen in Figure 20A treated by excision of the humeral head and insertion of a hemiarthroplasty.

ing an area of decreased sensation in the 'badge patch' area at the point of the shoulder.

Diagnosis

An antero-posterior and lateral or axial radiograph of the shoulder are required. The bone fragments may be impacted into each other or widely displaced. The greater and lesser tuberosities may form separate fragments and the humeral head may appear 'capsized' in the joint (Fig. 20A). Coexisting dislocation of the shoulder joint rarely occurs.

Management

Intracapsular fractures with marked displacement of the fragments may lead to avascular necrosis of the head. In these cases, a hemiarthroplasty is used (Fig. 20B). The stem of the prosthesis is fitted down the shaft of the humerus and the rotator cuff and greater and lesser tuberosities secured around its head. Early mobilisation of the shoulder is important to prevent the joint becoming stiff.

Impacted fractures of the surgical neck of the humerus are usually rested for a few days in a collar and cuff sling and pendulum exercises begun early in order to avoid shoulder stiffness.

Complications

Complications can involve:

- Early — axillary nerve palsy
- Late — frozen shoulder
  — malrotation.

2.4 **Femoral neck fractures**

A fracture of the femoral neck is the most common frac-

ture seen in the elderly female and usually occurs in the eighth and ninth decade of life. The cause is usually a simple fall at home but it may be associated with another medical problem, such as a stroke, hypotensive crisis or poor vision. Whatever the cause, the result may be the ultimate loss of independence, especially for someone who was previously just managing to live alone safely.

Classification

- intracapsular fractures occur within the capsule and may be transcervical or subcapital
- extracapsular fractures occur outside the capsule and may be sited through the base of the femoral neck (basal) or through the trochanters (intertrochanteric).

Why is it so important to differentiate intracapsular fractures from extracapsular fractures? Figure 21 shows the blood supply to the femoral head, which comes through the diaphyseal vessels along the femoral neck, via the foveal artery to a small area of the articular surface and, most importantly, via the retinacular vessels, which are reflected from the capsule along the femoral neck to enter the head around its margin. If these vessels are damaged by significant displacement from a subcapital fracture then avascular necrosis of the femoral head will result.

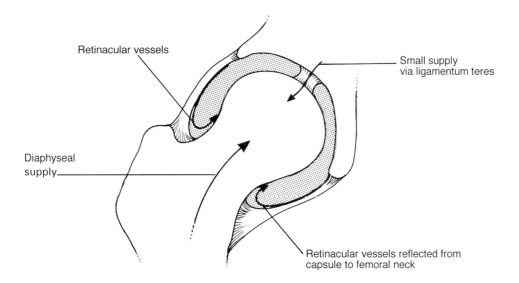

Retinacular vessels

Small supply
via ligamentum teres

Diaphyseal
supply

Retinacular vessels reflected from
capsule to femoral neck

Fig. 21
Blood supply to the femoral head.

Clinical features

- Listen — a usual history of the event is that of a frail old lady who has fallen at home and been found by neighbours after she has been lying on the floor all night. Apart from pain at the hip, the patient is often confused and may be suffering from hypothermia.
- Look — the affected leg is shortened and externally rotated.
- Feel — tenderness over the greater trocanter
- Move — pain on attempting movement of the hip.

A variety of medical problems are often present.

Intracapsular fractures

Diagnosis

An antero-posterior and lateral radiograph of the femoral neck are required (Fig. 22). If the line of the cortex of the medial side of the femoral shaft is traced upwards towards the pelvis it can be seen how this line continues along the inferior side of the neck of the femur until it comes to a sudden stop at the fracture site. The fracture in this case is intracapsular and in particular a subcapital fracture. If the fracture were not there, the line traced along the medial side of the shaft of the femur and the inferior side of the femoral neck would continue in a smooth curve along the inferior side of the superior pubic ramus (Shenton's line). A break in continuity of this line helps to find a fracture in the femoral neck (Fig. 23).

Management

Initial management includes rehydration, pain relief (often by skin traction to the affected leg) and treatment of underlying medical conditions.

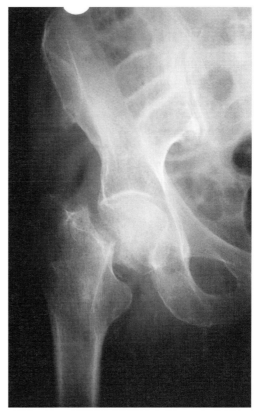

Fig. 22
Intracapsular (subcapsular) fracture of the femoral neck.

The natural history of a subcapital fracture is eventually avascular necrosis of the femoral head. However, this predicted sequel is pre-empted by prosthetic replacement of the femoral head at the time of injury. An uncemented hemiarthroplasty or a bipolar arthroplasty is used unless the patient is particularly active or young, when internal fixation should be attempted in an effort to preserve the patient's own hip.

Complications

Avascular necrosis of the femoral head is the main complication arising from an intracapsular fracture. Other complications may occur after hemiarthroplasty;

- dislocation
- erosion of acetabular floor
- need for revision surgery.

Extracapsular fractures

In Figure 24, observe how the fracture line passes obliquely through the greater trochanter at the top left of the picture across towards the lesser trochanter. This is an extracapsular fracture. This fracture is distal to the capsule and is sited through the trochanters at the base of the femoral neck.

Management

General medical management is required initially as it is for intracapsular fractures.

Extracapsular fractures would unite without treatment, but malunion would be present unless the external rotation and shortening were corrected. Traction could be used to prevent this, but the prolonged period of bed rest involved would give rise to many other complications which together would probably be fatal. For this reason the fracture is usually treated by closed reduction and fixed with an internal fixation device such as the dynamic hip screw. The barrel and sliding

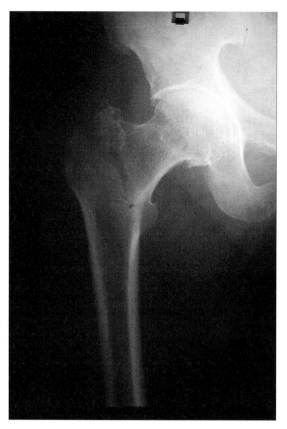

Fig. 24
Extracapsular (intertrochanteric) fracture of the femoral neck.

screw portion are positioned in the neck and head of the femur with radiographic screening using an image-intensifier. The plate is then secured to the upper femoral shaft by screws.

The patient can begin weight-bearing within 2 or 3 days of surgery and the screw will thus retract into the barrel as the fracture impacts. With this device, the patient has the best chance of regaining mobility and independence and of returning home.

Complications

Complications of prolonged bed rest include:

- pressure sores
- hypostatic pneumonia
- urinary tract infection
- disuse osteoporosis
- deep venous thrombosis
- pulmonary embolus.

Complications of internal fixation include:

- general complications of surgery
- implant failure
  — cutting out
  — breaking
- fracture through the porotic bone at the end of the plate.

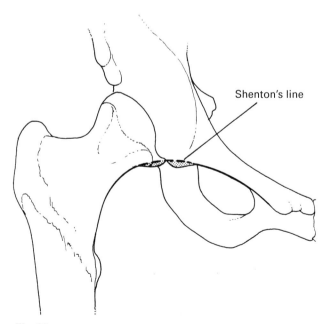

Fig. 23
Normal appearance of Shenton's line. Compare this with the radiograph of the fracture of the femoral neck in Figure 22.

Shenton's line

2.5 **Vertebral body fractures**

Patients with osteoporosis may suffer spontaneous vertical compression fractures of the vertical bodies. The thoracic vertebrae are most commonly affected but the lumbar vertebrae may also be involved.

Clinical features

An elderly lady gives a history of sudden onset of back pain after merely stooping or lifting a light object. Often there is a history of multiple similar events and, as a result, an increasing kyphosis becomes apparent in the thoraco-lumbar spine.

Characteristically, there are no neurological deficits in the limbs as there is no impingement of the spinal cord or nerve roots. The fractures are stable.

Diagnosis

Crush fractures of vertebrae characteristically form wedge shapes compressed anteriorly when seen on the lateral radiograph (Fig. 25).

Management

Symptoms are relieved by a short period of bed rest. Mobilisation should be recommended as soon as possible.

Complications

• increasing kyphosis
• pressure sores over the prominent spinous processes.

2.6 **Pathological fractures**

Pathological fractures occur through areas of abnormally weak bone.

Classification
Bone may be weak because of:

• generalised disease
  — myelomatosis
  — osteoporosis
  — osteomalacia and rickets
  — Paget's disease
• local disease
  — metastatic tumour
  — primary tumour
  — fibrous dysplasia
  — bone cysts.

The most common tumour seen in the skeleton is a metastasis from a primary tumour elsewhere. Usual sites of the primary are:

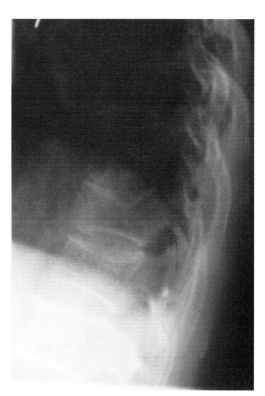

Fig. 25
Both wedge-shaped and bi-concave compression fractures are seen in the lower thoracic vertebrae in this woman with osteoporosis.

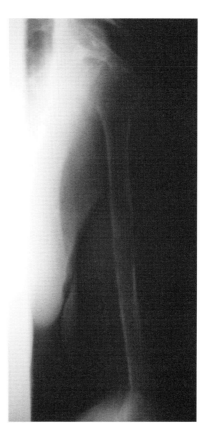

Fig. 26
Pathological fracture in the humerus in a patient with a primary breast carcinoma.

27

- bronchus
- breast
- prostate
- thyroid
- kidney.

Clinical features

The key features of a pathological fracture are:

- pain at the site, which pre-dates the injury
- a fracture caused by minimal trauma.

Diagnosis

Pathological fractures are characteristically transverse and may be widely displaced (Fig. 26).

Management

The local management of pathological fractures of long-bones usually require open reduction, curettage and fixation of the fragments, often with an intramedullary rod and cement. Postoperative radiotherapy controls pain and any micrometastases. The general management includes further investigation to find an occult primary tumour and to control it.

Complications

- hypercalcaemia
- dehydration
- occult primary
- second deposit elsewhere.

Self-assessment: questions

Multiple choice questions

1. Recognised complications of Colles' fracture include:
   a. Median nerve compression
   b. Loss of full supination
   c. Loss of dorsiflexion
   d. Sudek's atrophy
   e. Avascular necrosis of the lunate

2. The following complications are associated with a fracture of the surgical neck of the humerus:
   a. Avascular necrosis of the humeral head
   b. Non-union of the greater tuberosity
   c. Axillary nerve damage
   d. Loss of abduction
   e. Non-union

Case histories

History 1

> An 86-year-old lady is admitted to hospital after being found lying on her kitchen floor overnight. A fracture of the femoral neck is suspected.

1. What clinical features would confirm the diagnosis?
2. Explain the need for hemiarthroplasty in the presence of a displaced subcapital fracture of the femoral neck
3. What further medical problems would be associated with this lady's history?

History 2

> A 65-year-old lady presents complaining of sudden exacerbation of back pain. She has had a chronic pain in the same area for some months but yesterday while bending forwards to pick up something from the floor the pain became sharp, severe and persisting. An examination found well-localised mid-thoracic tenderness and a marked kyphosis at the site.

1. What is the clinical diagnosis?
2. What underlying pathology should be suspected?

> Radiological examination shows the suspected fracture to be through an area of lytic bone destruction.

3. What investigations would be appropriate in the further management of this patient?

Picture question

The radiograph (Fig. 27) shows a fracture through abnormal bone.

1. Indicate the fracture line
2. In what ways is the bone different from the opposite side in shape, size, density and architecture?

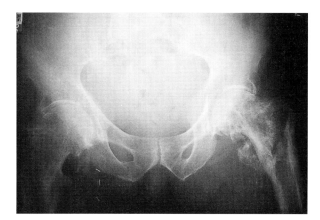

Fig. 27

Short notes

1. List three possible ways in which a Colles' fracture can be immobilised after reduction has successfully been achieved.
2. What would be the effect of prolonged bed rest on an elderly lady with a fractured femoral neck?

Viva questions

1. What is the most commonly seen skeletal tumour?
2. Damage to the axillary nerve is associated with what injury?
3. How would a patient be examined to confirm the integrity of axillary nerve function?

Self-assessment: answers

Multiple choice answers

1. a. **True.** Median nerve compression is sometimes seen as a complication of a displaced Colles' fracture. Bony fragments or haematoma compress the median nerve in the carpal tunnel. It is not seen in the majority of cases in elderly patients. However, if compression is suspected, carpal tunnel decompression should be carried out early.

   b. **True.** Full supination may be lost as a result of malunion of a Colles' fracture. The distal fragment is displaced into pronation and unless corrected will not rotate normally into full supination as the distal radio-ulnar joint moves.

   c. **False.** The distal fragment in a Colles' fracture is displaced dorsally so loss of dorsiflexion is not seen in cases of malunion. However, palmar flexion may be lost as the normal arc of motion of the wrist joint is displaced dorsally. After reduction of a Colles' fracture, there may be residual stiffness of the wrist, causing some loss of dorsiflexion.

   d. **True.** Although some stiffness, pain and swelling may persist after treatment of a Colles' fracture, a full-blown Sudek's atrophy is rare. In these cases there is pain, swelling, stiffness in the hand and wrist, which is sweaty and cold.

   e. **False.** Avascular necrosis of the lunate (Keinbock's disease) is an uncommon condition affecting the lunate. It occurs spontaneously. The aetiology is unclear.

2. a. **False.** A fracture of the surgical neck of the humerus does not interrupt the blood supply to the humeral head. Avascular necrosis is not, therefore, seen.

   b. **False.** A fracture of the surgical neck is below the tuberosities.

   c. **True.** The axillary nerve winds round the neck of the humerus to supply the deltoid muscle and a small area of skin over its insertion onto the humerus.

   d. **True.** Damage to the axillary nerve associated with the fracture results in paralysis of the deltoid and loss of abduction.

   e. **False.** Fractures of the surgical neck of the humerus unite readily.

Case history answers

History 1

1. Clinical features would include tenderness over the greater trochanter and loss of movement on the affected side. The injured leg lies in external rotation and is shorter than the opposite side.

2. A hemiarthroplasty is used in the treatment of displaced subcapital fractures when avascular necrosis of the femoral head can be assumed to be inevitable. An Austin–Moore hemiarthroplasty or a bipolar arthroplasty are used.

3. A person who has been lying on the floor all night is likely to have developed hypothermia. Signs of this should be specifically sought and treatment instituted.

History 2

Picture answer

1. There is an intertrochanteric fracture line through the abnormal bone.

2. The bone is larger, more bent and of varied density compared with the opposite side. The cortex is thin and the normal medullary architecture is lost. The radiograph is of a pathological fracture through an area of Paget's disease in the bone.

Short notes answers

1. A variety of methods of splinting a Colles' fracture are available. Minimally displaced and stable fractures are usually treated in a below-elbow plaster cast. Unstable and comminuted fractures may require stabilisation with percutaneous wires or with an external fixator.

2. Prolonged bed rest for an elderly lady would carry a high morbidity and can be fatal. Complications of this form of management would include:

   * pressure sores
   * hypostatic pneumonia
   * deep venous thrombosis
   * urinary tract infection
   * further osteoporosis.

Viva answers

1. Skeletal metastases from breast, bronchus, prostate, thyroid or kidney primaries.

2. The nerve is in jeopardy in fractures of the neck of the humerus.

3. The axillary nerve innervates the deltoid muscle and causes abduction of the shoulder. It supplies sensation to the 'badge patch' area over the point of deltoid insertion.

Fractures in children

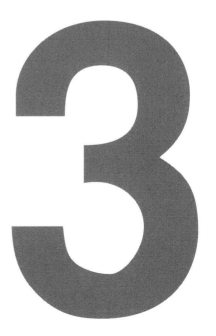

3.1 Clinical examination

A gentle and friendly approach are always required when examining children. Care must be taken not to cause any additional pain. Fracture sites must always be palpated very gently and any movement likely to cause pain carried out cautiously and slowly. An initial temporary splint or sling is comforting and after this has been applied it is usually possible to check the presence of peripheral circulation and sensation without causing more discomfort. On examining injuries around the elbow, much information can be gained by comparing the injured with the non-injured site, paying particular attention to the carrying angle. A radiograph of the uninjured elbow can be useful, but the parent's permission to X-ray the uninjured side must always be sought and the reason explained.

When interviewing the family of a child with a skeletal tumour or in whom you suspect non-accidental injury, great sensitivity must be exercised to avoid causing unnecessary grief or hostility.

Fracture patterns

Because the growing bone has not yet fully ossified, skeletal injuries are different from those seen in adults.

The bones are less brittle (more plastic) than those of adults. A moderate force will cause a child's bone to buckle on the compression side. With more force the distraction side of the bone will fracture causing the classical 'greenstick' fracture (Fig. 28A). The growth plate of the bone (the physis) has not yet fused and continues to separate the epiphysis from the metaphysis (Fig. 28B). Through this area particular injuries have been recognised.

Epiphyseal injuries. These injuries take place through the calcifying layer of chondrocytes in the epiphyseal plate or physis.

Salter and Harris described various types of epiphyseal injury (Fig. 29).

Slipped lower radial epiphysis

Clinical features

A fall on the outstretched hand in a child is the common presentation of this injury. Dorsal swelling and deformity are obvious.

Diagnosis

Careful examination of a lateral radiograph is necessary to detect posterior displacement of the epiphysis and to identify any associated fracture in the metaphysis or epiphysis.

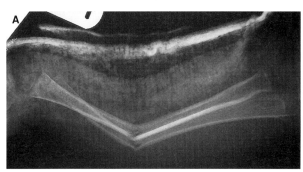

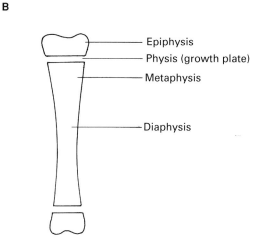

Fig. 28
Greenstick fracture **A.** Fracture of both bones of the forearm. The compression side is still intact but the fracture is present through the cortex on the opposite side of the bone. **B.** The immature skeleton grows longitudinally by the action of the growth plate situated between the epiphysis and the metaphysis.

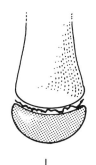 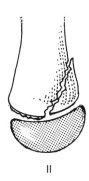 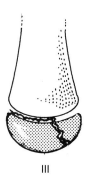 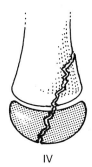 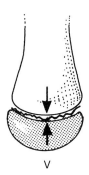

I   II   III   IV   V

Fig. 29
Salter and Harris classification of epiphyseal injuries. I—The injury has separated the epiphysis from the metaphysis through the growth plate. II—The injury passes through a corner of the metaphysis. This is the most common injury. III—The injury passes through the epiphysis itself. IV—The fracture line crosses the physis from epiphysis to metaphysis. This type of injury can result in premature fusion of the epiphysis to the metaphysis. V—There has been a compression force on the physis. The radiograph appears normal.

Management

Gentle, accurate manipulation under anaesthesia is required to reduce the fracture and avoid damaging the blood supply to the epiphysis. Open reduction is occasionally indicated but if internal fixation is required only fine wires should be placed across the physis as mechanical disturbance may cause premature fusion of the epiphysis and growth arrest.

Complications

* premature epiphyseal growth arrest
* median nerve compression.

Slipped upper femoral epiphysis (SUFE)

Clinical features

Patients are usually boys. Classically two types of patient present with this condition. One is an athletic adolescent with sudden onset of hip pain often occurring at sports. The other is characteristically hypogonadal and overweight with a gradual history of pain usually involving both hips.

* Listen — pain is often referred to the knee.
* Look — the leg is externally rotated and appears short (Fig. 30).
* Feel — local tenderness
* Move — internal rotation is resisted.

Diagnosis

Careful examination of an antero-posterior radiograph and comparison with the opposite side, if this is not affected, shows the displacement of the femoral head. Lateral radiographs and other specially angled views will show the extent of the posterior slip of the head on the neck more clearly (Fig. 31).

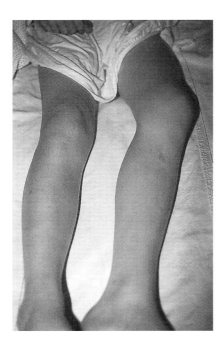

Fig. 30
This 15-year-old presented with sudden pain in the left hip after a sporting event; the leg is externally rotated and shortened.

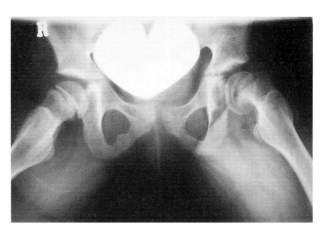

Fig. 31
The radiograph of the pelvis shows the capital epiphysis has slipped off the femoral neck on the left side. On the right side there is a suggestion of an early slip.

Management

Manipulation of the slipped epiphysis runs the risk of causing avascular necrosis of the head. Pinning of the capital epiphysis in the slipped position is, therefore, favoured. In cases of severe slip, an osteotomy of the femoral neck can be planned later.

Complications

* avascular necrosis
* chondrolysis, which later causes osteoarthritis.

3.2 Forearm fractures

Because of their structural immaturity, children's bones are more plastic than adult bones. Consequently, when subjected to bending forces such as those occurring in a fall on the outstretched hand, they suffer plastic deformation rather than a break.

In some cases, the bone only buckles on the compression side (torus fracture). In other cases, the cortex breaks on the distraction side of the bone and bends on the compression side (greenstick fracture, see Fig. 28A).

Clinical features

Fractures of both the bones of the forearm is a common injury in children. Falls from a height or from a bicycle are often the cause.

* Listen — the injured limb is painful
* Look — the fracture site is swollen, bruised and deformed.
* Feel — peripheral circulation and sensation may be compromised by compression of the neurovascular bundles by the displaced fracture or the resulting swelling (Fig. 28A).
* Move — movement is restricted and rotational deformity may be apparent.

Diagnosis

Two radiographs at right angles to each other are required to assess fully the extent of the fracture. The amount of displacement, angulation or rotation at the fracture site can be assessed. Complete displacement at the fracture site results in overriding of the bones' ends, causing shortening.

Management

Manipulation under anaesthetic is required to correct the deformity. The fracture is immobilised in the reduced position by an above-elbow plaster cast.

During the following few days, the limb must be carefully observed for signs of acute compartment compression, which may develop as a result of the injury or of the manipulation. Pain in the forearm aggravated by passive extension of the fingers suggests that the deep muscle bellies are compressed within their fascial compartment. Peripheral sensation and circulation may be impaired. Emergency treatment consists of releasing all constricting dressings. If this does not relieve the symptoms, an extensive surgical decompression of the two forearm compartments by incision of the skin and deep fascia is required. These wounds are left open for 2 to 3 days before attempting delayed primary closure or covering with a split thickness skin graft.

Complications

- acute compartment syndrome
- median nerve compression
- malunion, causing loss of rotation.

3.3 Elbow fractures

Supracondylar fractures

This injury is an orthopaedic emergency as a delay in treatment may cause irreversible forearm ischaemia by pressure on the brachial artery. The median nerve also may be compressed or injured.

Clinical features

- Listen — a fall from a bicycle or a swing onto the outstretched hand in a young child is the usual presentation.
- Look — there is deformity and bruising at the elbow and a tense swelling develops quickly (Fig. 32).
- Feel — the radial pulse must be palpated and if weak or absent the elbow should be gently extended to minimise any kinking of the brachial artery in the ante cubital fossa. Symptoms and signs of medial nerve compression may be apparent in the hand, and

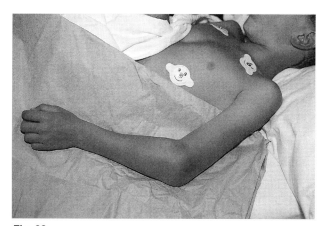

Fig. 32
Supracondylar fracture of the elbow of an 8-year-old boy.

rarely the ulna and radial nerves may be affected too.
- Move — all elbow movements are resisted.

Diagnosis

An antero-posterior radiograph shows varus or valgus angulation at the fracture site but a lateral view looks the most dramatic especially in completely displaced fractures (Fig. 33A). The distal fragment is displaced posteriorly in nearly all cases.

Management

It is usually possible to correct the displacement by manipulation under anaesthetic. The reduced position is checked by axial and lateral radiographs. The reduced position is maintained by full elbow flexion, which locks the distal fragment in place by tensioning the triceps aponeurosis posteriorly. If accurate reduction is not possible by closed means, then open reduction is required to visualise the fracture and secure it in an anatomical position with Kirschner wires (Fig. 33B).

Complications

- early complications:
  — acute occlusion of the brachial artery
  — median nerve damage
  — compartment syndrome
- later complications:
  — Volkmann's ischaemic contracture
  — myositis ossificans
  — malunion.

Fractured lateral condylar mass

Avulsion fractures of the lateral aspect of the humerus may produce a displaced fragment that may be rotated and, therefore, impossible to reduce by closed means (Fig. 34A).

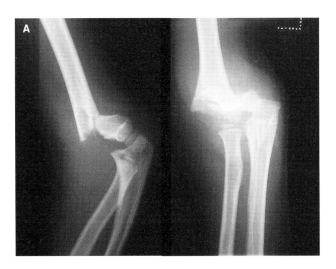

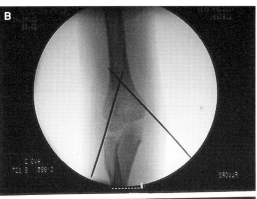

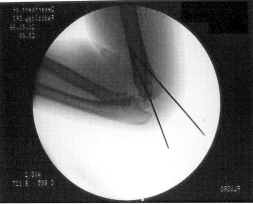

Fig. 33
Supracondylar fracture. **A.** Radiograph showing gross displacement at the fracture site. The associated kinking and compression of the brachial artery and median nerve can be imagined as they pass anterior to the bone fragments. **B.** Kirschner wires used to secure a supracondylar fracture in the reduced position.

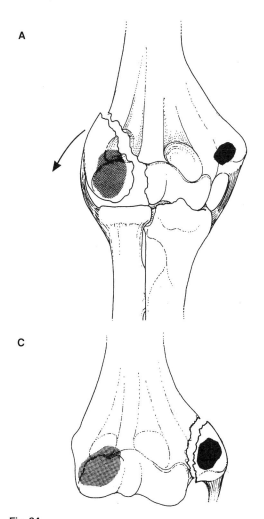

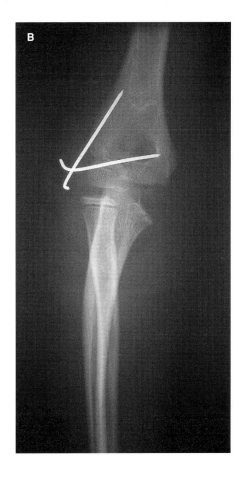

Fig. 34
Fracture of the lateral condylar mass. **A.** Diagram showing the mechanism of rotation and displacement caused by the fracture. **B.** Kirschner wire fixation of the fracture seen in (A). **C.** A fracture of the medial epicondyle may displace so that the fragment lies within the joint.

Diagnosis

The radiograph may be difficult to interpret if one is not familiar with the normal pattern of the centres of secondary ossification around the elbow. A comparison radiograph of the uninjured elbow is often helpful.

Management

Accurate reduction by operative exposure and securing the fragment with a suture or Kirschner wire produces a secure anatomical position (Fig. 34B).

Complications

- non-union
- development of valgus deformity as a result of premature growth arrest
- tardy ulnar palsy.

Medial epicondylar avulsion

A valgus injury to the elbow may avulse the medial epicondyle (Fig. 34C). Sometimes it is only slightly displaced but on other occasions it is widely separated and becomes trapped in the joint space.

Diagnosis

Careful comparison of the radiograph with that of the non-injured elbow makes it easier to recognise the displaced epicondyle.

Management

Anatomical reduction usually requires an open procedure with fixation of the avulsed epicondyle by a Kirschner wire.

Complications
- pressure on the ulnar nerve
- premature epiphyseal growth arrest causing varus deformity of the elbow with growth.

3.4 Femoral fractures

Clinical features

Direct trauma, often from being knocked down by a vehicle, accounts for the majority of femoral fractures in children. On examination, the affected leg is shorter, swollen and externally rotated. There may be considerable blood loss into the tissues.

Diagnosis

Although the diagnosis is apparent clinically, a radiograph is necessary to assess the fracture pattern and the degree of displacement and angulation.

Management

Prompt fluid replacement is required to avoid cardiovascular collapse, but care must be exercised in young children to avoid circulatory overload. Fractures in young children can be managed in gallows traction for 3 to 4 weeks until healing occurs (Fig. 35), but older children require skin traction, usually on a Thomas splint.

Complications

- shock
- nerve or vessel injury
- malunion
- leg length discrepancy.

3.5 Dysplasia, tumour and non-accidental injury

Fractures in children in the absence of significant injury raises the possibility of bone dysplasia, tumour or non-accidental injury. If a fracture is not apparent on the radiograph in the painful area, it must be scrutinised carefully to look for any periosteal elevation. This is

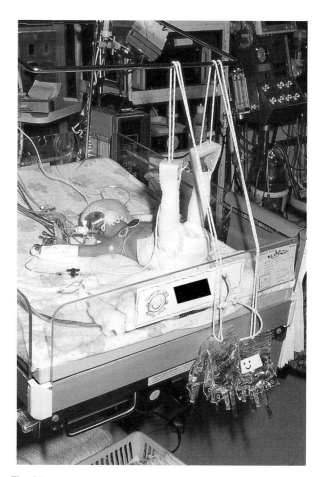

Fig. 35
Gallows traction being used to manage a femoral fracture in a neonate.

seen as a thin calcified line above the cortex and is caused by elevation of the periosteum by:

- blood from a crack in the cortex
- a subperiosteal haematoma
- pus
- tumour.

Dysplasia

Fibrous dysplasia. The bone is soft and weak with extensive areas of fibrous tissue. Fractures and deformity develop.

Osteogenesis imperfecta. There is often a positive family history, but occasionally a case occurs as a result of a new mutation. A spectrum of severity can occur from multiple fractures, causing deformity and stunted growth, to mild cases with only discoloured sclerae or joint laxity.

Management

- simple immobilisation of fractures
- prevention of more fractures
- early discharge after hospital treatment.

Complications

- decreased growth
- progressive deformity
- multiple fractures.

Tumour

Bone tumours may be benign or malignant.

Bone cyst. A bone cyst is an apparent space in the medullary cavity surrounded by thinned cortex containing solid, uncalcified material. Radiographically the appearance suggests a tumour. However, it is benign and may resolve spontaneously if a fracture occurs through it.

Other tumours:
- enchondroma
- aneurysmal bone cyst

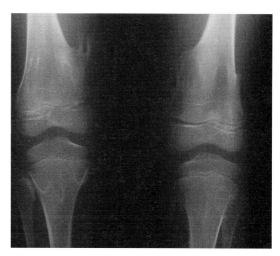

Fig. 36
Multiple exostoses around the knees of a 6-year-old child. They characteristically appear to grow away from the epiphysis.

- multiple exostoses (Fig. 36)
- malignant bone tumours (occur rarely).

Non-accidental injury

This must be suspected in any child if there seems to be parental indifference to the injury and if no reasonable explanation for the fracture is given. Particular vigilance is necessary with very young children who are unable to speak for themselves. Other features that support this diagnosis are:

- fractures at a variety of stages of healing
- soft tissue injuries
- depressed attitude of the child
- indifferent or aggressive attitude of the parents.

Management

- admit to hospital
- skeletal survey
- paediatrician
- social worker.

Self-assessment: questions

Multiple choice questions

1. A boy aged 12 presents with pain and a limp in the right leg of 2 months' duration. Likely diagnosis includes:
   a. Late presentation of congenital dislocated hip
   b. Transient synovitis of the hip
   c. Perthes' disease
   d. Acute septic arthritis
   e. Slipped femoral epiphysis

2. When managing fractures in children:
   a. The presence of multiple fractures of different ages is pathognomonic of non-accidental injury (NAI)
   b. The presence of pain on passive extension of the toes after a closed tibial fracture is due to impingement of the muscle bellies at the fracture site
   c. Failure to achieve a satisfactory reduction round the elbow warrants open reduction and internal fixation
   d. Conservative treatment is used less frequently than internal fixation for the stabilisation of femoral shaft fractures
   e. The initial treatment of impending compartment syndrome would be the release of all constricting plaster bandages

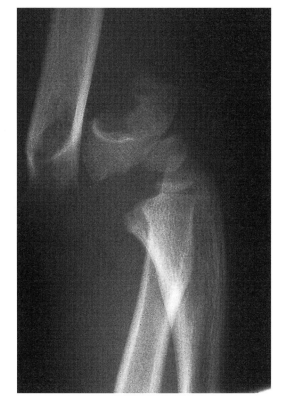

Fig. 37

Case history

An 8-year-old child presents with a painful, swollen and bruised elbow after a fall from a swing.

1. What structures in the area are in jeopardy from a fracture in this area?
2. Look at Figure 37. What is the injury? In what position would you put the arm to restore peripheral circulation?
3. Discuss the complications of non-anatomical reduction of this fracture

Picture questions

Picture 1

Study the elbow radiograph of a 6-year-old boy in Figure 38 and answer the following questions.

1. What is the name of this injury?
2. How should the injury be managed?
3. What complications may result?

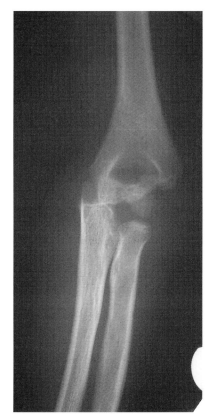

Fig. 38

Picture 2

Figure 39 shows the radiograph of a wrist of a 7-year-old boy who has fallen from his bicycle. You can see the epiphyseal plate is still open in this growing child. Look carefully at the lateral radiograph.

1. Identify the distal radial epiphysis and classify the type of injury.

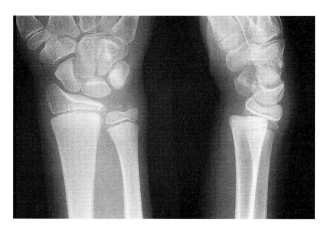

Fig. 39

Essay questions

1. Discuss the conditions that should be considered by the incidental finding of periosteal elevation on the radiograph of a child's tibia.
2. List the clinical findings that suggest the development of an acute compartment syndrome.

Viva questions

1. How would you manage a child who you suspect is a victim of non-accidental injury?
2. How would you treat a 2-year-old child with a femoral shaft fracture?

Self-assessment: answers

Multiple choice answers

1. a. **False**. A case of congenital dislocation of the hip (CDH) missed on routine screening in infancy would have presented early in childhood when the patient began walking. It is unlikely that the first presentation of CDH would be as late as the age of 12.

   b. **False.** Transient synovitis of the hip has a short duration and usually resolves within 3 to 4 days.

   c. **True.** Perthes' disease develops spontaneously, causing pain and limp that may persist for episodes of several weeks. Symptoms are relieved by rest but recurrent relapses are characteristic until the area of avascular necrosis heals.

   d. **False.** Acute septic arthritis is characterised by acute severe pain in the hip and loss of movement.

   e. **True.** A gradual slip of the upper femoral epiphysis presents with a prolonged history of pain and loss of movement. The condition is associated with hormonal imbalance in the adolescent. Acute slips have a shorter history and may be associated with direct trauma.

2. a. **False**. The child may have bone dysplasia such as osteogenesis imperfecta. Other features such as bruising are required to make the diagnosis of NAI.

   b. **False.** The presence of pain on passive extension of the toes in this case is caused by ischaemia of the muscle bellies and not by impingement at the fracture site. The findings suggest impending compartment syndrome.

   c. **True.** In general, operative techniques and anaesthetic procedures are now so safe and reliable that it is in the patient's best interests to change the fracture management to open reduction and internal fixation if a satisfactory position cannot readily be achieved or held by conservative measures.

   d. **False.** Conservative treatment is the usual method of splinting femoral shaft fractures in children.

   e. **True.** Compartment syndrome is suspected by the presence of intractable pain in the limb exacerbated by passive extension of the digits. There may be associated paraesthesia or numbness in a peripheral nerve distribution. If symptoms are not relieved by releasing all constricting dressings, fasciotomy should be undertaken sooner rather than later.

Case history answer

1. The structures most in jeopardy following an elbow fracture are the brachial artery, median nerve and ulnar nerve.

2. The radiograph shows a displaced supracondylar fracture in this child. Peripheral circulation can be restored by splinting the elbow in extension to minimise kinking of the brachial artery.

3. Complications of non-anatomical reduction of this fracture will be rotatory malalignment or varus or valgus angulation of the forearm at the fracture site.

Picture answers

Picture 1

1. The radiograph shows the avulsion of the medial epicondyle.

2. Management of this injury requires anatomical reduction of the fragment. This may require an open procedure if the medial epicondyle is displaced and trapped within the joint (Fig. 40).

3. Failure of anatomical reduction and fixation may result in the development of premature epiphyseal growth arrest causing various deformities of the elbow.

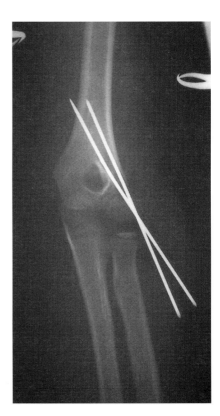

Fig. 40. Kirschner wire fixation of the displaced fracture of the medial epicondyle.

Picture 2

1. The lateral radiograph shows posterior displacement of the epiphysis, which has taken a small wedge of the dorsal metaphysis with it. This is the common Salter Harris type II injury.

Essay answers

1. The presence of periosteal elevation suggests the presence of pus, blood or tumour between the bone cortex and periosteum. Investigation should be aimed at looking for a occult fracture in the cortex and a subperiosteal haematoma. The presence of infection should be eliminated by white cell count and plasma viscosity. A CT scan or MRI scan may be helpful in diagnosing a tumour.
2. The presence of compartment syndrome is recognised by pain on passive extension of the digits. There may be peripheral congestion, swelling and discoloration of the digit. Sensation is impaired.

Viva answers

1. A child in whom you suspect non-accidental injury should be admitted to hospital for observation. A skeletal survey is carried out to detect the presence of fractures at various stages of healing. A thorough clinical examination is required to detect the presence of soft tissue injuries. Help from the paediatrician and the social work department are required before the discharge of the child to a place of safety or back home can be arranged.
2. A young child with a fractured shaft of the femur is best managed in gallows traction. Elastoplast bandages secure cords to the ankle that are attached to weights at the foot of the bed. The hips are flexed to 90° and sufficient weights added to elevate the buttocks slightly from the mattress. Nursing care is facilitated in this position and the weight of the child's body provides counter traction to the fracture site. Within 3 or 4 weeks the fracture will have healed.

Orthopaedic disorders of children

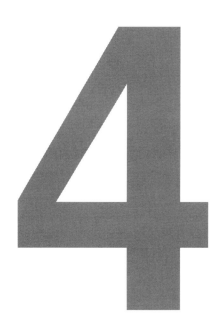

4.1 Clinical examination

Before examining children it is important to have gained their confidence by friendly conversation or play and to avoid any sudden or potentially painful actions. It is important that the examination is carried out in a warm environment and that the doctor has warm hands. The examination is almost impossible if the child becomes unsettled or distressed because of your initial approach.

Examine the patient walking, standing and lying.

Walking. Observe for an antalgic gait or a Trendelenburg gait.

Standing. Observe the contour of the lumbar spine, the posture of the pelvis and whether the feet are flat on the floor. The presence of calcaneovalgus and associated flat foot should be observed. Flexion of the spine by asking the patient to touch the toes will unmask and exaggerate any scoliosis.

Lying. Put the hips through a full range of movement; internal rotation particularly is limited if there is a synovial effusion in the hip joint, and any movement of the hip will be impossible in the presence of acute septic arthritis. When examining a neonate for congenital dislocation of the hip (CDH) remember that Ortolani's and Barlow's tests must be carried out gently to avoid causing vascular damage to the capital epiphysis. With the patient sitting on the couch carefully examine the foot and ankle. Three movements should be elicited: ankle movement, which is pure flexion and extension, subtalar movement, which involves moving the os calcis into inversion and eversion, and midtarsal joint movement, which includes internal and external rotation.

4.2 Minor disorders

Children with minor or transient conditions are frequently referred to paediatric orthopaedic clinics because parents are worried that a serious abnormality may be developing.

In-toeing. Parents complain that their toddler is always tripping over his feet. Examination should exclude three common abnormalities which cause the leg or foot to rotate inwards: femoral neck anteversion, tibial torsion and metatarsus adductus. Usually each of these causes is self-limiting and is unlikely to require intervention.

Knock knee. Normal physiological development of the lower limbs shows a progression from genu varus in the first 2 years of life through normal alignment at the age of 3 to genu valgus with a characteristic gap between the malleoli at the age of 4 (Fig. 41).

Flat feet. Postural or mobile flat feet are common in children and are caused by physiological ligamentous laxity, which disappears with age. The medial fat pad in

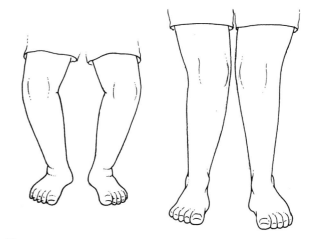

Fig. 41
During the first years of life a child's knees change from a genu varus position through normal alignment to a genu valgus position by the age of 4 years.

the sole of the foot exaggerates the appearance. Calcaneus valgus is seen when the feet are viewed from behind but the heel corrects to normal alignment and the medial arch reappears when the child stands on tip toe. Rigid or spastic flat foot is much rarer and is caused by an underlying abnormality of the tarsal bones and associated muscle spasm.

4.3 Irritable hip

A common cause of unwillingness to weight-bear or of limping in a child is a transient synovitis of the hip. This condition, as its name suggests, is a self-limiting inflammation of the joint lining resulting from synovial irritation. As such it is quite benign. However, several other diagnoses should be excluded:

* acute septic arthritis
* Perthes' disease.

Irritable hip can be due to:

* idiopathic causes
* recent upper respiratory tract infection
* minor trauma.

Clinical features

* Listen — history of recent intercurrent illness
* Look — the leg lies in mild external rotation
* Feel — typically there is tenderness
* Move — there is limited movement of the joint. Internal rotation is especially limited because this movement has the effect of tightening the joint capsule and so constricting the effusion even further and increasing the pain.

Diagnosis

Investigations are directed to eliminating the other possible causes of hip pain. An X-ray of the hip is taken to look for features of Perthes' disease (Fig. 42).

A white cell count and plasma viscosity are used to exclude a diagnosis of septic arthritis.

A throat swab and ASO (antistreptolysin O) titre may help to confirm a recent upper respiratory tract infection.

Management

After a short period of bed rest, the child's symptoms usually settle. There are no long-term complications but the child may have another similar episode in the future.

4.4 Osteochondritis

Osteochondritis occurs in several locations and is usually caused by a transient interruption of the blood supply to an area of growing bone; the mechanism by which this occurs is unknown.

Perthes' disease

Boys between the ages of 5 and 10 years are usually affected. There is a recurring history of episodic pain in the hip, which causes a limp and limitation of movement. Internal rotation and extension are particularly affected.

Diagnosis

Radiographs show sclerosis and irregularity of the capital epiphysis (Fig. 42). Sequestration may be apparent and the head may be flatter than normal and appear to be extruding from the acetabulum.

Management

Treatment is aimed at *containing* the hip while maintaining movement. An abduction splint may be required

but in milder cases limitation of activities during exacerbation of symptoms is sufficient. In severe cases where the femoral head has extruded from the acetabulum a femoral neck osteotomy is required to relocate the head in the acetabulum.

Other sites of osteochondritis

Osteochondritis dissecans. The lateral side of the medial femoral condyle is the usual site for an area of avascularity to develop. An island of bone demarcates and eventually may separate and become a loose body in the joint, causing intermittent locking and pain in the knee (see p. 104).

Traction apopyhysitis. Osgood–Schlatter's disease is a common example of a traction apophysitis. Idiopathic aseptic necrosis of the tibial tuberosity causes knee pain in adolescence which is usually exacerbated by vigorous activity. The tibial tuberosity is elevated and tender. Radiographs show elevation, sclerosis and fragmentation of the tuberosity and, in older patients, a fragment of bone is sometimes seen in the patellar tendon. Management consists of avoiding sports when symptoms are severe. Sometimes a splint or plaster cylinder is used to enforce this (Fig. 43).

Kienbock's disease. This condition presents in young adults with pain and stiffness of the wrist caused by avascular fragmentation and collapse of the lunate. Radiographs show increased density.

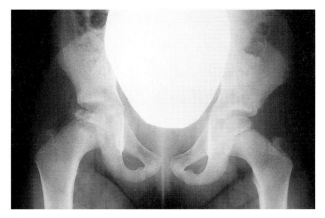

Fig. 42
Perthes' disease of the right hip compared to the opposite normal side. The capital epiphysis is flattened, sclerotic and fragmented.

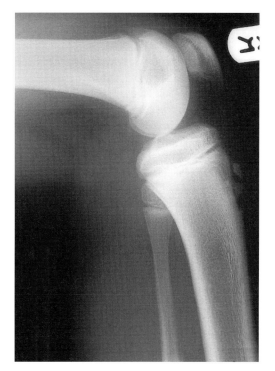

Fig. 43
Osgood–Schlatter's disease. The tibial tuberosity is elevated, sclerotic and fragmented.

4.5 Congenital hip dysplasia

Opportunities to examine babies for possible congenital dislocation of the hip (CDH) are available in postnatal wards, paediatric clinics, the paediatric orthopaedic service and general practice. Although the quoted incidence of CDH is only between one and two per 1000 live births, the consequences of missing a case are severe and distressing for the child and the parents.

Predisposing factors are:

- family history
- developmental factors — intrauterine malposition, breech presentation
- environmental factors — swaddling.

Clinical features

- Listen — positive family history, difficult birth
- Look — asymmetrical buttock creases. Short leg or Trendelenburg gait when standing. If bilateral there is a characteristic waddling gait
- Feel — the hip may be felt to relocate during manipulation
- Move — there is loss of full abduction of the hips in flexion, a 'click' or 'clunk' noise may be heard from the hip while changing a nappy.

If the diagnosis is not made until adult life, the presentation is of hip pain, resulting from secondary osteoarthritis, and the presence of a positive Trendelenburg sign.

Diagnosis

Ortolani's and Barlow's tests are most commonly used in the neonatal period (Fig. 44). In Ortolani's test a 'clunk' sound and the sensation of the hip relocating can be elicited while the hip is gently manipulated into flexion and abduction. The sensation and sound are quite different from the physiological soft tissue 'click' often heard from the hip in the natal period.

Radiographs do not show the capital epiphysis in the first months of life but it can be visualised by ultrasound or arthrography. Radiographs at the age of 9 months, however, can be used to predict the position of the capital epiphysis and to measure the acetabular angle. Von Rosen views are used to predict whether the joint is dislocated (Fig. 45).

Management

If the diagnosis is made in the first 2 months of life, then effective treatment can be instituted early. This involves holding the hips in abduction and flexion in a von Rosen splint (Fig. 46) or Pavlic harness.

After the age of 2 months a period of traction and plaster immobilisation will be required.

By the age of 12 to 18 months, open reduction is nec-

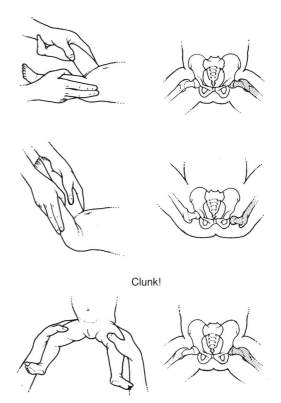

Clunk!

Fig. 44
Ortolani's test (see text for description).

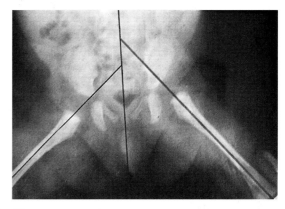

Fig. 45
A von Rosen view radiograph of the hips taken with the legs internally rotated. The long axis of the femur should point through the triradiate epiphysis if the hip is in joint.

essary to remove limbus and capsule which may be blocking anatomical reduction. A subsequent derotation osteotomy is often required as the hip is only stable in the reduced position if fully internally rotated.

Complications
Complications arising from failure to make an early diagnosis include:

- persisting limp
- hip pain
- later osteoarthritis.

Complications that can occur as a result of treatment include:

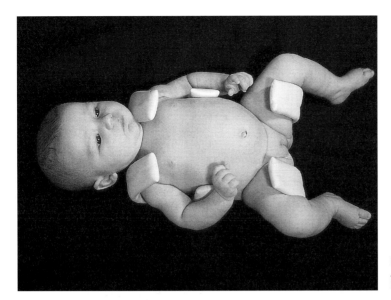

Fig. 46
A von Rosen splint used to keep the dislocated hip in the reduced position.

- avascular necrosis of the femoral head
- recurrent dislocation.

4.6 Infection

Once a serious and common illness, bone and joint infection in childhood is now only rarely seen in westernised countries. Vigilance, however, is more important to ensure that a case is not missed, and the possibility of infection must always be considered in the differential diagnosis of any patient with joint pain or limp.

Acute osteitis

The metaphyseal area of a long bone is the usual site of acute osteitis and often the proximal tibia is the location. There may be a history of minor trauma to the area, which causes a small haematoma. Bacteraemia from a remote infective source colonise this and produce an abscess which may discharge onto the skin or, if the epiphysis is within the joint capsule, into the joint itself, causing septic arthritis.

Clinical features

- Listen — there is intense pain at the site involved
- Look — the child is unwell with a pyrexia and sweating
- Feel — the infected area is tender, hot, swollen and red. A subperiosteal abscess may be palpable
- Move — any movement of the joint is resisted.

Diagnosis
Blood tests show positive blood cultures, elevated ESR (erythrocyte sedimentation rate) or plasma viscosity, and a polymorphonuclear leucocytosis. In later stages, radiographs will show an elevation of the periosteum.

Management
Conservative treatment begins with elevation of the limb to reduce pain. After all investigations are under way, the 'best-guess' antibiotic can be commenced. This is usually a combination of fucidic acid and flucloxacillin, as the organism usually responsible is *Staphylococcus aureus*. Occasionally *Haemophilus influenzae* is isolated, in which case amoxycillin or co-trimoxazole are indicated. If the symptoms fail to settle surgical exploration and drainage of the area is required.

Complications

- Brodie's abscess — an interosseus collection of pus which repeatedly becomes symptomatic
- chronic osteitis — characterised by sinus, sequestrum, involucrum and growth arrest.

Septic arthritis

A joint may become infected from adjacent osteitis, bacteraemia or a penetrating wound into the joint. Left untreated progressive bacterial destruction of the articular cartilage will occur.

Clinical features
The child is unwell and pyrexial. The joint is swollen, tender to touch and inflamed. Movement is resisted.

Diagnosis
White cell count, blood culture and plasma viscosity measurements are all required. Radiological examination is unlikely to be helpful.

Management
Early commencement of 'best-guess' antibiotics is necessary. Although *Staphylococcus aureus* is the most likely organism, gonococcal infection should not be forgotten. It may be necessary to open the joint to aspirate pus for bacteriological examination and to set up irrigation. Accessible joints can be treated by arthroscopy (see p. 104).

Complications

- secondary osteoarthritis
- spontaneous ankylosis
- chronic osteitis.

4.7 Talipes equinovarus

Congenital talipes equinovarus (TEV) in its severest form is an uncommon condition. There may be a positive family history. The condition is characterised by failure of development of the postero-medial muscles of the calf and also of the os calcis and forefoot.

A milder more commonly seen condition is postural TEV, which results from the position of the fetus in utero.

Clinical features

The affected foot is held in equinus and varus and cannot be corrected passively by manipulation (Fig. 47). In severe cases, the calf muscles seem small and the os calcis is underdeveloped.

Diagnosis

The diagnosis is easily made on clinical examination, but failure to start treatment promptly may compromise a satisfactory result.

Management

Within the first 6 weeks of life, manipulation of the foot by the mother can stretch out the deformity and this will be entirely effective in patients with pure postural TEV. More severe cases may require subsequent elastoplast strapping or plaster of Paris splinting.

If correction has not been achieved by the age of 6 weeks, a postero-medial release of the Achilles tendon, flexor hallucis longus and flexor digitorum longus will be required. After the age of 5 years, bony abnormalities are established and a wedge of tarsal bones must be removed from the lateral side to enable the foot to be put in a plantigrade position on the ground.

Complications

- incomplete correction
- rocker-bottom foot — due to failure to correct the equinus hindfoot aspect of the deformity
- small foot — even when corrected there will still be loss of normal development of the foot.

4.8 Scoliosis

Although uncommon, it is necessary to be able to recognise the presence of scoliosis as missed cases may

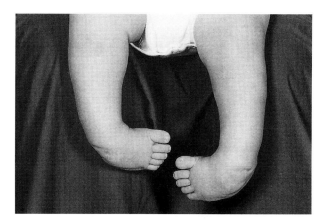

Fig. 47
Bilateral talipes equinovarus.

progress to produce severe cosmetic deformity. Scoliosis is excessive spinal curvature in a coronal plane. It can be classified as postural or structural. Structural scoliosis may have varying causes:

- idiopathic
- congenital
- neuromuscular
- miscellaneous.

Idiopathic scoliosis is the most common variety and it is more common in girls than in boys.

Clinical features

The cosmetic deformity of a thoracic curve, usually convex to the right, is reported as an incidental finding by the family. The degree of deformity becomes progressively severe during adolescence until growth ceases. Forward flexion exacerbates the deformity. In later stages, secondary osteoarthritic degeneration in the spine may cause pain and stiffness.

Diagnosis

Radiology confirms the diagnosis by showing the presence of rotated vertebrae. The degree of curve is classically measured as the angle between the end plates of the normal vertebrae above and below the abnormal section (Cobb's angle) (Fig. 48).

Management

Because cases only present rarely it is best if management of all but the mildest curves is carried out in regional specialist spinal centres. Plaster of Paris immobilisation has been recommended for infantile idiopathic scoliosis but this condition may resolve spontaneously with time. The role of corrective orthoses has probably been overstated in the past and is now less popular.

Extensive corrective spinal surgery is carried out in progressive, severe disease with dramatic results but at

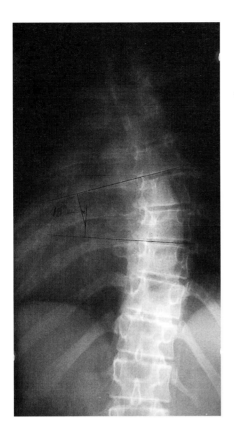

Fig. 48
A mild thoracic scoliosis with a Cobb's angle of 15 degrees.

the risk of the considerable complications of implant failure or even spinal cord damage.

Complications

- progression of the curve and development of a rib hump
- secondary osteoarthritis
- cardiopulmonary embarrassment in progressive cases starting in infancy.

Self-assessment: questions

Multiple choice questions

1. The following are possible sequelae of acute osteitis:
   a. Looser's zones found on radiograph
   b. sequestrum formation
   c. septic arthritis
   d. fracture of the affected bone
   e. myositis ossificans

2. In congenital dislocation of the hip (CDH):
   a. Abduction in flexion is limited
   b. The acetabulum fails to develop normally
   c. The femoral head is displaced posteriorly on the femoral neck
   d. Forceful manipulation may precipitate avascular necrosis of the head
   e. Reduction may be blocked by the ligamentum teres

3. Talipes equinovarus:
   a. Is associated with CDH
   b. Necessitates tendon transfer in its management
   c. Necessitates repeated and frequent reviews
   d. Is associated with dislocating patellae
   e. Certain types respond to simple manipulation and splinting

Case history

A teenage sportsman complains of pain in the knee getting worse since training increased. The symptoms have persisted for 3 weeks and now cause limping. There is local tenderness at the tibial tuberosity but no swelling and no hotness.

1. What is the most likely diagnosis?
2. What radiographic findings are associated with this condition?
3. What treatment would you recommend?

Picture question

Figure 49 shows the feet of a 2-year-old child.

1. What features can be observed?
2. What manoeuvre would the child be asked to carry out while you observe the feet?
3. What is the diagnosis and what management should be recommended?

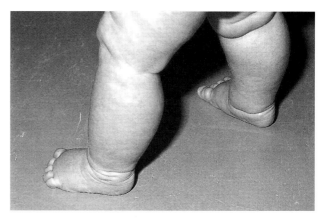

Fig. 49
Feet of a 2-year-old child.

Short notes

1. Transient synovitis is often a diagnosis of exclusion. What investigations would help you to exclude a diagnosis of septic arthritis which may present in a similar way?
2. Describe the investigations used to diagnose CDH.

Viva questions

1. Describe how you would examine and investigate a teenage girl presenting with scoliosis.
2. What are the principles behind the early management of CDH?

Self-assessment: answers

Multiple choice answers

1. a. **False.** Looser's zones are associated with osteomalacia.
   b. **True.** A portion of cortex may lose its blood supply as a result of the surrounding infection and become sequestrated as an island of dead bone.
   c. **True.** Osteitis in the metaphysis may spread to involve the adjacent joint, if the area of infection is within the joint capsule.
   d. **True.** The architecture of the infected bone is less strong than normal bone.
   e. **False.** Myositis ossificans is associated with calcification of an intramuscular haematoma and is, therefore, associated with fractures particularly around the elbow.

2. a. **True.** The dislocated hip resists full abduction in flexion. This is demonstrated by Ortolani's test.
   b. **True.** The absence of the femoral head within it causes the acetabulum to develop as a shallow recess rather than in the normal shape.
   c. **False.** In CDH there is no abnormality of the alignment of the femoral head on the neck. This configuration is seen in slipped upper femoral epiphysis.
   d. **True.** During relocation of a dislocated hip, the blood supply to the femoral head may be jeopardised causing avascular necrosis of the bone or cartilage.
   e. **True.** Several soft tissue structures at the hip may block reduction of a CDH. The ligamentum teres is one such structure.

3. a. **True.**
   b. **False.** Initial management depends on manipulation and splintage. Later lengthening of the Achilles tendon and medial tendons is required.
   c. **True.**
   d. **False.**
   e. **True.** Postural talipes equinovarus responds well to simple manipulation and splinting while the more severe types associated with underdevelopment of the calf and os calcis usually require early surgery.

Case history answer

1. The history of anterior knee pain at the tibial tuberosity associated with sports in a teenager suggests a traction apophysitis rather than an infective lesion. The teenager probably has Osgood–Schlatter's disease.

2. The lateral radiograph will sometimes show a small avulsed portion of the tongue of the tibial apophysis or occasionally a separate ossicle, but the latter is usually seen in an older patient.

3. Having a rest from sports will relieve the acute symptoms and this can be enforced with an above-knee splint. The symptoms characteristically relapse and remit until the lesion heals.

Picture answer

1. The medial longitudinal arches of this toddler's feet cannot be seen. There is calcaneus valgus deformity.

2. Asking the patient to stand on tip-toe will reconstitute the longitudinal arch and correct the valgus alignment of the heels.

3. This is a case of postural flat foot. No particular treatment is indicated but support for the shoe heels may help to prevent them from deforming and wearing down so quickly.

Short notes answers

1. A plasma viscosity and white cell count would be the first-line investigations to institute in the case of a child with a limp. If the results are normal or only slightly raised, a diagnosis of acute septic arthritis is unlikely.

2. The following investigations may be used to diagnose CDH. Before the age of 9 months, the capital epiphysis is not visible radiologically but the cartilaginous head can be outlined by the intra-articular injection of contrast medium. This will show the configuration of the joint and whether the head is subluxated or not. A less invasive investigation is an ultrasound scan, but the findings are difficult to interpret.

   In a child over the age of 9 months, a plain X-ray of the pelvis may give some indication as to whether the head of the femur is likely to be in joint or not. Acetabular angle may indicate whether the acetabulum is likely to be dysplastic or normal, and von Rosen views are used to predict whether the joint is dislocated.

Viva answers

1. The patient's spine must be observed from behind and any scoliosis or rib hump noted. Asking the patient to touch the toes will exacerbate the deformity. Postural scoliosis resulting from leg length inequality is neutralised when the patient's back is observed when sitting down. Radiographs of the spine are used to visualise the deformity and calculate the angle of the curve (Cobb's angle).

2. The principles of management of CDH are to contain the head within the acetabulum so as to allow normal development of each to precede. Manipulation must be gentle and immobilisation of the reduced hip must not be rigid.

Backache and neckache

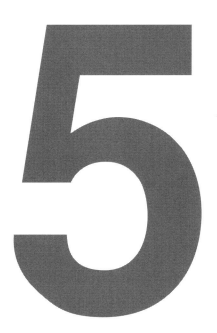

5.1 **Clinical examination**

Examination includes both a local examination of the axial skeleton and a neurological examination of the limbs.

Local examination

Cervical spine. Observe any abnormal posture of the neck and the presence of muscle spasm. Localised tenderness can be elicited with one-finger palpation of the vertebral spines. Full range of flexion, extension, lateral flexion and rotation should be attempted.

Lumbar spine. The patient should be examined standing. The lumbar spine is observed from behind and from the sides for loss of the normal lumbar lordosis and the presence of paravertebral muscle spasm. Full range of spinal extension, flexion and lateral flexion and rotation should be elicited. Pain associated with spinal extension classically suggests facet joint or posterior column pathology, while pain associated with forward flexion suggests intervertebral disc or anterior column pathology. A patient with sciatica often stands with a scoliosis to one side in an attempt to relieve traction on the compressed nerve root.

Neurological examination

In cervical spondylosis and brachalgia, observation of the arms may show muscle wasting. Areas of altered sensation should be sought by careful examination in each dermatome. Muscle weakness and diminished reflexes should be sought.

Patients with sciatica should be examined lying supine. The legs are observed for muscle wasting. Sensation is examined in a dermatome pattern and weakness or diminished reflexes elicited. Exacerbation of pain by straight leg raising should be sought in both legs.

With the patient prone, sensation in the sacral dermatome can be tested by examining perianal sensation. In all cases of disc prolapses, a rectal examination should be carried out to detect any loss of normal anal tone suggestive of a central disc prolapse. The femoral nerve stretch test, which involves extension of the hip, can also be attempted in this position.

If time allows, additional examination for the inappropriate signs associated with functional overlay can be attempted.

5.2 **Mechanical back pain**

Backache is the cause of many hours lost from work and many visits to orthopaedic departments. The vast majority will be due to a mechanical backache and only a small minority will result from prolapse of an intervertebral disc or other specific abnormality.

Clinical features

Patients complain of acute onset of back pain, which may radiate to the buttock and knee on the affected side but not any further. There is a history of some heavy lifting or of a long period of sitting with the spine in a flexed position such as when driving a car. There are no neurological deficits on examination of the legs.

Diagnosis

Radiological examination is unremarkable but an incidental finding of some disc space narrowing and an occasional osteophyte may be seen. However, the radiographs must be carefully scrutinised for the presence of an occult tumour, usually a metastasis from a primary bronchial, breast or renal tumour. Any questionable areas must be further investigated by CT scan.

Management

Management of mechanical back pain involves:

* rest until the initial symptoms settle
* analgesics
* heat and gradual spinal extension exercises
* lumbosacral support (this sometimes helps)
* learning correct posture and lifting techniques.

Surgery for back pain is usually inappropriate.

Complications

Patients' interpretation of their symptoms may be complicated by:

* functional overlay
* an outstanding claim for compensation which complicates management.

5.3 **Nerve root entrapment**

Prolapsed intervertebral disc

The lumbar disc is composed of the annulus fibrosus, which surrounds the nucleus pulposus. As the disc loses its water content as part of the degenerating process, the annulus fibrosus softens, allowing the nucleus pulposus to bulge posteriorly towards the spinal canal. Compression of a nerve root may result. Extruded fragments of degenerate disc may become lodged in a nerve root canal (Fig. 50).

Clinical features

Patients complain of the local effects of pain in the back and of lower motor neurone symptoms in the legs.

* Listen — pain is more severe in the leg than the back and radiates to below the knee. In classical sciatica, pain is felt on the dorsum of the foot in the dermatome distribution of L5 or S1

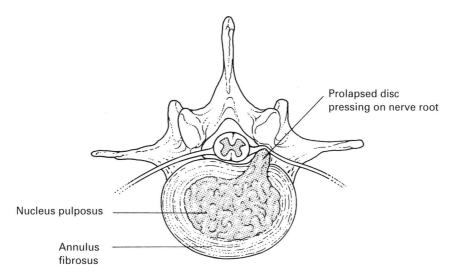

Fig. 50
Pressure on a lumbar nerve root due to herniation of the nucleus pulposus through the annulus fibrosus of the intervertebral disc.

- Look — examination of the spine shows spasm in the paravertebral muscles, loss of lumbar lordosis and possibly scoliosis at the involved level
- Feel — sensation may be diminished in the dermatomes supplied by the involved spinal nerves (Fig. 51)
- Move — straight leg raising is diminished, tendon reflexes may be absent or depressed and power is weakened in the appropriate myotomes.

Patients with a central disc prolapse may develop urinary retention and a neurogenic bladder from compression of the sacral nerve root of the cauda equina. Physical examination shows loss of anal tone and perianal anaesthesia.

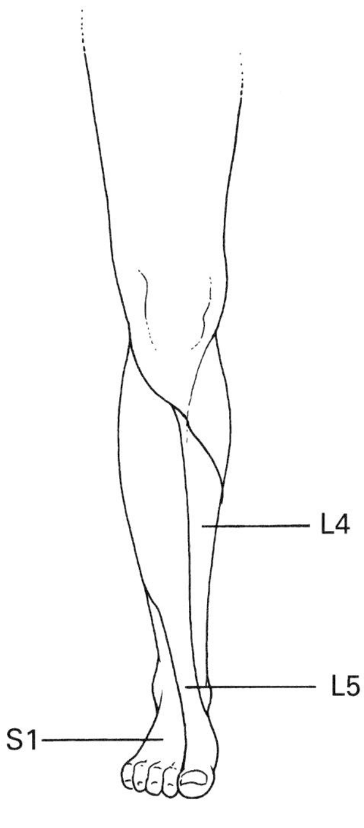

Diagnosis

Injection of radio-opaque contrast material into the spinal canal (radiculography) outlines the nerve roots and shows the site of compression. L4/5 and L5/S1 are the most frequently affected levels for disc prolapse. CT or MRI scan may also visualise the site of root compression (Fig. 52).

Management

Cauda equina lesions need emergency decompression if permanent bowel and bladder dysfunction are to be avoided.

Fig. 51
Dermatome distribution in the lower limb.

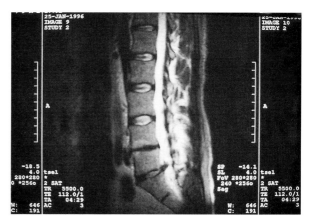

Fig. 52
MRI scan showing posterior prolapse of the disc at L5/S1.

The majority of the remaining cases, however, will settle as the disc shrinks again with a period of bed rest. Traction, analgesia and muscle relaxants may help the patient to conform to these restrictions. Disc excision by fenestration of the lamina is required for patients for whom conservative treatment fails or who are in severe pain. Microdiscectomy under operating microscope control has more recently been used to minimise the morbidity associated with more extensive surgery.

Complications

- persisting back pain
- interfacet joint degeneration
- arachnoiditis
- missed diagnosis of spinal tumour.

Other causes of nerve root entrapment

Two conditions must be considered:

- bony nerve root entrapment
- spinal stenosis.

Bony nerve root entrapment

In bony nerve root entrapment, there is impingement of an osteophyte on a spinal nerve root in the root canal (Fig. 53).

Clinical features
Usually the patient is older than those with prolapsed intervertebral disc. There is pain in a dermatome distribution but, in addition, there is an ill-defined pain from osteoarthritic degeneration of the facet joints. Pain is usually less severe than with prolapsed intervertebral discs.

Diagnosis
Plain radiographs and CT scan, together with contrast enhancement, will help to identify the site of nerve root compression.

Management
Simple methods of local pain relief are used initially. In selected patients, decompression of the nerve root canal may help.

Spinal stenosis

Even a mild degree of osteophytosis will cause impingement in the spinal canal if this is already narrow. In such patients, a minor degree of congestion in the spinal canal produces symptoms.

Clinical features
Exercise-induced pain in the buttocks and legs, especially when walking, gives rise to the description of symptoms as 'spinal claudication'. Symptoms are exacerbated by standing and extending the spine and relieved by sitting and flexing.

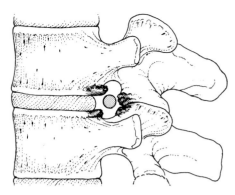

Fig. 53
In bony nerve root entrapment the spinal nerve is compressed by osteophytosis from the adjacent joints.

Diagnosis
A narrow spinal canal can be diagnosed from the CT scan.

Management
Weight reduction and limitation of activities that involve extension of the spine may help. Laminectomy is required in some patients to decompress the spinal cord.

Complications

- arachnoiditis
- missed diagnosis of spinal tumour
- spinal instability after laminectomy.

5.4 **Spondylolisthesis**

There are several causes of spondylolisthesis, but the underlying abnormality in them all is a forward slip of one vertebra on another, usually of L5 on S1, caused by a defect in the pars interarticularis, the part of the vertebrae between the superior and inferior articular facets.

Different types of spondylolisthesis include:

- dysplastic
- isthmic
- degenerative
- traumatic
- pathological.

The isthmic type is the most common.

Clinical features

The patient is classically a young active person who complains of low back pain radiating to the buttocks. On examination, a step may be felt in the tender area at the base of the lumbar spine.

Diagnosis

Oblique radiographs are required and show either a lucent area in the pars interarticularis or a slip of one vertebrae on the other at this point (Fig. 54).

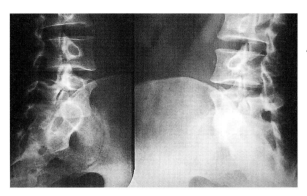

Fig. 54
Oblique radiograph showing a spondylolisthesis at L4 but without any forward slip of the vertebrae.

Management

Rest during acute episodes, a spinal support and extension exercises may all help. A lumbo-sacral fusion is indicated for progressive slips.

Complications

- persisting back pain.

5.5 **Ankylosing spondylitis**

This uncommon inflammatory disease affecting young males between the ages of 15 and 30 years is part of a complex multijoint disease.

Clinical features

There is stiffness in the lumbar spine and low back pain. There is often a positive family history. In severe cases of the disease, gross flexion and fusion of the entire spinal column is seen and chest wall expansion becomes limited. Other joints may also be involved.

Diagnosis

Radiological examination in patients presenting early shows fusion of the sacro-iliac joints. Eventually the characteristic 'bamboo spine' develops.

Management

Rest and non-steroidal anti-inflammatory analgesics followed by mobilisation are aimed to keep the patient's spine as mobile and comfortable as possible.

Complications
In addition to the natural progression of the conditions, other systems can be involved:

- colitis
- uveitis.

5.6 **Tumours and infection**

Tumours

Metastases must always be considered in cases of undiagnosed pain in the back. The usual primary sites are:

- prostate
- breast
- kidney
- bronchus.

Osteoblastoma, giant cell tumour and multiple myeloma are examples of primary bone tumours that may be seen; primary spinal canal tumours such as neurofibroma and meningioma are also occasionally encountered.

Clinical features
There is localised back pain, possibly of long duration, that is severe and unrelenting. Root signs may be absent.

Diagnosis
Metastatic deposits are seen as lytic lesions on plain radiographs and are usually sited in the pedicles of the vertebrae. Unlike the other metastases, prostatic metastases can also be sclerotic. A myelogram or MRI scan will demonstrate a spinal canal tumour (Fig. 55).

Management
Management involves decompression and radiotherapy.

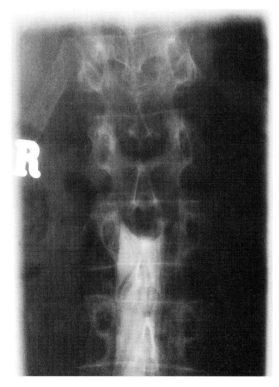

Fig. 55
Neurofibroma in the spinal canal demonstrated by a lumbar myelogram.

Complications

- vertebral collapse
- nerve root invasion
- spinal cord compression resulting in paraplegia.

Infection

Patients with acute infective discitis are usually elderly or immunosuppressed. Spread of infection may involve an adjacent vertebra. Tuberculous discitis is rare in westernised countries.

Clinical features

Severe back pain is present but pyrexia may be absent. Plasma viscosity and ESR are elevated, but the expected leucocytosis is absent.

Diagnosis

A needle biopsy will retrieve pus for bacteriological examination but sometimes an open biopsy is required.

Management

High doses of 'best-guess' antibiotics are required while laboratory results are awaited. Spontaneous intervertebral fusion tends to occur when the infection is cured.

Complications

- kyphosis
- spinal cord compression.

5.7 Cervical spondylosis

Cervical spondylosis is the name given to chronic degeneration of the cervical spine involving the intervertebral discs and the ligamentous and osseous structures associated with them. It can be responsible for a spectrum of problems ranging from mechanical neck pain to cervical cord compression.

Figure 56 shows the normal anatomical relationship between the intervertebral foramen and the two adjacent vertebral bodies. The intervertebral disc lies anteriorly and the facet joint posteriorly. The emerging nerve root is shown end-on.

Figure 57 shows how degeneration of the cervical disc and the associated osteophyte formation around the vertebral end-plates can press on the nerve roots and on the spinal cord itself. With increasing age, the intervertebral disc loses its water content and shrinks. In doing so, its height decreases and movement at the interfacet joints is altered. Osteoarthritic degeneration of these joints can then occur.

Radiological evidence of degeneration of the cervical discs is seen in 50% of the population over the age of 50 and 75% of the population over the age of 65. However, this may be an incidental finding and the patient may have no symptoms. However, if the spinal canal measures less than 13 mm on CT scan its contents

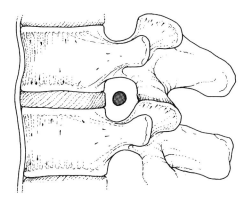

Fig. 56
Normal anatomical relationship between the intervertebral foramen and the two adjacent vertebral bodies. The nerve root exits through the intervertebral foramen.

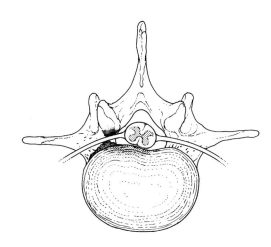

Fig. 57
Compression of the spinal nerve root and the cord itself following cervical disc degeneration and associated osteophytosis of the adjacent joints.

are more at risk from compression and symptoms will ensue.

Acute cervical disc prolapse is uncommon (unlike lumbar disc prolapse). Severe trauma to the cervical spine is necessary to produce this injury. When it occurs, it is usually in young patients. More commonly, cervical disc herniation is an acute-on-chronic phenomenon seen in older patients.

The following syndromes are associated with cervical spondylosis:

- mechanical neck pain
- radiculopathy
- myelopathy.

Mechanical neck pain

This is the most common presentation of cervical spondylosis.

Clinical features

- Listen — neck pain and associated muscle spasm originating from facet joint degeneration radiates to the occiput and shoulders but there is no pain radiating down the arms. Symptoms are worse with activity and in the morning.
- Look — the neck may be held to one side
- Feel — localised tenderness in the paravertebral muscles
- Move — there is only slightly decreased range of movement in the cervical spine because 50% of rotation takes place at the atlanto-axial joint, which is not usually affected.

Management

The majority of patients respond to simple treatment. A cervical collar may provide a comfortable support. Heat treatment, cervical traction and non-steroidal anti-inflammatory analgesics may all be tried. In the majority of patients, however, the symptoms will settle with time.

Radiculopathy

Clinical features

Radiculopathy is the name given to the symptoms produced when a nerve root is compressed by or stretched around an osteophyte or prolapsed intervertebral disc. The settling down of one facet joint on another following shrinking of the intervertebral disc causes narrowing of the intervertebral foramen, which also contributes to compression on the nerve root. Patients complain of lower motor neurone symptoms in the arms.

- Listen — patients complain of pain in a dermatome distribution in the arm (brachalgia) (Fig. 58)
- Look — wasting of the muscles in the myotome involved
- Feel — there may also be decreased sensation in the appropriate dermatome
- Move — Muscle weakness and depressed tendon reflexes.

Diagnosis

An oblique radiograph will show encroachment of osteophytes at the intervertebral foramen. More detail will be gained by an MRI scan or a cervical myelogram (Fig. 59).

Management

Conservative

- cervical collar
- cervical traction
- analgesics.

Surgical. When conservative measures fail, decompression of the compressed nerve root by excising the adjacent osteophytes (see below) can be carried out electively.

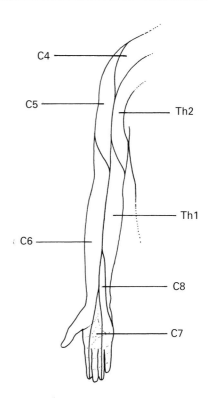

Fig. 58
Pattern of dermatomes in the upper limb.

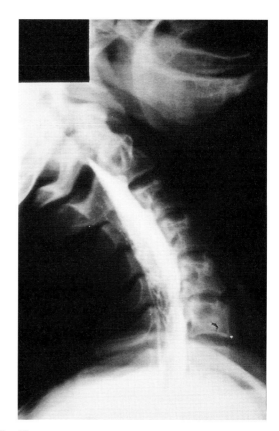

Fig. 59
Cervical myelogram showing indentation of the contrast medium by osteophytes at C5/6.

Myelopathy

Clinical features

Pressure from a protruding cervical disc or the associated osteophytes may cause pressure on the spinal cord itself. This is present when patients exhibit upper motor neurone signs in the legs and lower motor neurone signs in the arms. Patients complain of the insidious onset of weakness, clumsiness and dysaesthesia in the hand and may develop difficulty in walking because of spasticity and weakness of the lower limbs and retention of urine due to a neurogenic bladder.

Diagnosis

Cervical myelogram or MRI.

Management

Surgical decompression is urgently required for patients who develop symptoms of cervical cord compression. In the classic operation of anterior cervical decompression, a core of vertebral body and intervertebral disc is drilled out and prolapsed material removed. Osteophytes can be trimmed through the same approach to decompress the spinal cord and the nerve root canal.

Self-assessment: questions

Multiple choice questions

1. In a 40-year-old patient with a prolapsed intervertebral disc affecting S1 root, the following signs and symptoms are classically found:
   a. Limited straight leg raising in the affected leg
   b. Absent knee jerk
   c. Absent ankle jerk
   d. Weakness of extensor hallucis longus
   e. Weakness of plantar flexion of the ankle

2. In cervical spondylosis:
   a. The majority of patients respond to conservative treatment
   b. Pressure on a cervical nerve root causes upper motor neurone signs to be present in the arms
   c. Assessment of the lower motor neurone deficits helps to identify the level of the cervical lesion
   d. Wasting of the interossei muscles in the hand suggests a C5/6 disc prolapse
   e. Unlike a prolapsed lumbar intervertebral disc, a prolapsed cervical disc does not merit surgical intervention

3. A man with a prolapsed lumbar intervertebral disc suddenly develops dribbling of urine. He requires:

   a. Traction applied to the leg that has the associated sciatica
   b. MRI scan
   c. Transuretheral resection of the prostate
   d. Urgent exploration and excision of the appropriate disc
   e. Two weeks of strict bed rest

Case history

A 58-year-old man consults his doctor complaining of a 4-week history of pain in the back of the neck extending over the left shoulder. The patient further describes pain in the radial border of his forearm. In this area, there is also decreased sensation.

1. What further findings would be expected to be present on physical examination?
2. What investigations would be helpful at this stage?
3. At which level would the cervical lesion be expected to occur?
4. How should the management of this patient proceed?

Picture question

Study the radiograph of the cervical spine (Fig. 60).
1. What condition is being demonstrated by this oblique view?
2. What condition is demonstrated by the radiograph of the lumbar spine of this young man (Fig. 61)?

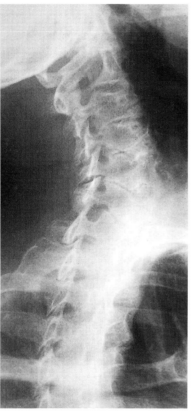

Fig. 60
Oblique view of the cervical spine.

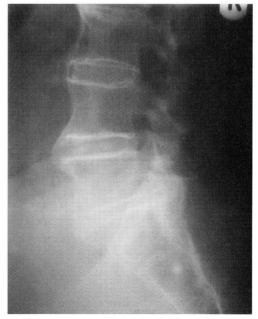

Fig. 61
Radiograph of the lumbar sacral region.

Short notes

1. Describe the radiological features of spondylolisthesis.
2. List the most likely primary sites of a neoplasm presenting with spinal metastases. Outline the key presenting features and the usual management of spinal metastases.

Viva questions

1. Demonstrate how to examine the back to elicit signs associated with a prolapse of the L5/S1 intervertebral disc.
2. In a patient complaining of backache and sciatica describe the features that are usually thought to be inappropriate clinical findings in the condition described in (Question 1) and indicative of functional overlay.

Self-assessment: answers

Multiple choice answers

1. a. **True.** Symptoms from S1 nerve root compression are exacerbated by traction on the nerve to which this root contributes. Stretching the sciatic nerve by flexing the hip with the knee fully extended, therefore, exacerbates the symptoms.
   b. **False.** The knee jerk is supplied by nerve roots L3 and 4. The ankle jerk is supplied by S1.
   c. **True.** The ankle jerk is absent as it is supplied by S1.
   d. **False.** Extensor hallucis longus is supplied by L5 and is, therefore, functioning.
   e. **True.** Plantar flexion of the ankle is controlled by S1 and is, therefore, weak.

2. a. **True**. In most patients, simple analgesics, heat, rest and sometimes longitudinal traction will relieve symptoms of cervical spondylosis.
   b. **False.** Pressure on a nerve root produces lower motor neurone signs, but if the cervical cord is compressed in the spondylitic process then upper motor neurone signs may be present in the lower limbs.
   c. **True.** The pain and paraesthesia in a particular dermatome will help to elicit the level of the cervical nerve root compression. The neurological level can be confirmed by looking for weakness or loss of tendon reflexes in the appropriate myotome.
   d. **False.** The interossei muscles are supplied by the T1 root and are, therefore, weak or wasted when the compression is at this level.
   e. **False.** In the presence of unremitting pain, progressive motor weakness or evidence of cord compression, surgical decompression at the appropriate level is required.

3. a. **False**. Although lumbar discs may shrink and resolve with conservative therapy, the presence of a central prolapse causing pressure on the sacral nerve roots manifesting itself by the presence of a neurogenic bladder requires urgent surgical decompression.
   b. **True.** The clinical diagnosis can be confirmed rapidly by MRI scan or lumbar myelogram.
   c. **False.** The dribbling incontinence is caused by a neurogenic bladder with retention and overflow and not by outlet obstruction.
   d. **True.** Urgent decompression of the involved nerve root is required.
   e. **False.**

Case history answer

1. The patient describes pain and the doctor detects diminished sensation in the area of the forearm corresponding to the dermatome supplied by the sixth cervical nerve root. Therefore, weakness of the wrist dorsiflexors, which are innervated by the same nerve root, would also be expected. The supinator reflex jerk may also be diminished.
2. An oblique radiograph of the cervical spine may show osteophyte encroachment on the nerve root between the sixth and seventh cervical vertebrae.
3. Compression of the C6 nerve root is expected.
4. If the patient's symptoms do not respond to conservative treatment, the presence of an objective finding of nerve root compression and of persisting pain would merit an anterior cervical decompression of the appropriate nerve root.

Picture answer

1. Nerve root entrapment at multiple levels can be seen on this oblique view which shows encroachment of bone into the neural foramen.
2. The radiograph shows the features of ankylosing spondylitis with calcification in the soft tissues around the lumbar spine.

Short notes answers

1. A oblique radiograph of the lumbar spine in spondylolisthesis will show a radiolucent defect across the pars interarticularis. When present, this finding appears like a collar on a bony shape resembling a 'scottie dog'. In patients where a slip has occurred at this area, there will be a step in the vertebral alignment between two adjacent vertebral bodies.
2. The most common primary tumours to metastasise to the skeleton are breast, prostate, kidney and bronchus. Patients complain of localised severe back pain present for a prolonged period without remission. There may be associated nerve root compression features. In these patients, surgical decompression is appropriate and radiotherapy to the area will relieve the local pain. For certain tumours (breast and prostate) chemotherapy may be strikingly effective.

Viva answers

1. With the patient standing, there may be loss of normal lumbar lordosis, muscle spasm in the paravertical muscles and loss of full flexion. Symptoms may be exacerbated by lateral flexion in one direction.

   Lying supine there may be obvious muscle wasting. Sensation will be diminished in the S1 dermatome on the lateral side of the lower leg and foot. There will be weakness of plantar flexion of the hallux. The ankle jerk is diminished or absent. Straight leg raising would be limited by pain.

2. Inappropriate clinical findings indicative of functional overlay include exacerbation of pain by axial loading of the skeleton, pain experienced by hip flexion but without the knee in extension and the ability to sit forwards on the examination couch while the legs are still fully extended.

Shoulder and elbow disorders

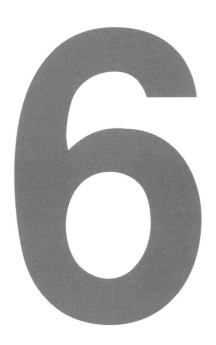

6.1 Clinical examination

Examination of the shoulder and elbow provides plenty of opportunity to exercise the routine of 'look, feel and move'.

Shoulder

Look. With the patient suitably undressed, the shoulders can be observed from all sides and compared. It is helpful to sit the patient down and observe the shoulders from above as well as from the front and sides. Loss of normal lateral contour is indicative of a dislocation of the shoulder or wasting of the deltoid. Scars, swelling and inflammation can also be looked for.

Feel. Bony outlines of the pectoral girdle can be felt beginning at the sternoclavicular joint, continuing along the clavicle to the acromioclavicular joint and tracing around the point of the acromion along the spine of the scapular. Finally the angle of the scapular can be palpated. The upper humerus and tuberosities may be felt in thin people. Tenderness over the joints can be noted.

Move. The full extent of flexion and extension is observed. When assessing abduction, the angle of the scapular should be immobilised to determine how much abduction is true glenohumeral movement and how much is scapulothoracic rotation. With the elbows tucked into the sides, external rotation and internal rotation can be noted. Because the abdomen gets in the way of internal rotation this movement can be further assessed by observing how far the patient can reach up their back with each hand.

Elbow

Look. An effusion in the elbow and swelling of the olecranon bursa are easily seen at the elbow. Rheumatoid nodules over the olecranon are common findings.

Feel. The bony prominences of the medial and lateral epicondyles and of the olecranon are readily palpable and form the points of an equilateral triangle. The radial head can be palpated and during pronation and supination of the forearm, crepitus may be felt here by the examining thumb.

Move. Any loss of full extension of the elbow can be measured and the range of flexion noted. Supination and pronation must be examined with the elbows stabilised against the chest wall to eliminate any contributory movements from the shoulder. Varus or valgus laxity of the elbow should be sought.

6.2 Shoulder disorders

Shoulder pain

Pain in the shoulder is a common complaint. It may be referred pain from the cervical vertebrae, radicular pain from cervical nerve root entrapment or intrinsic pain caused by specific pathology in the shoulder joint itself.

Acute supraspinatus tendonitis

This condition is seen in young adults and occurs commonly. Inflammation of the supraspinatus muscle in the rotator cuff produces a swollen area on the rotator cuff which becomes squashed beneath the acromion during abduction.

Clinical features

- Listen — there is sometimes a history of unaccustomed heavy use of the shoulder prior to the onset of symptoms
- Look — patients prefer to keep the shoulder still
- Feel — there is tenderness over the anterior rotator cuff
- Move — initially abduction is comfortable, but between 30 and 60 degrees it becomes painful; beyond 60, however, when the inflamed portion of the rotator cuff advances beyond the tight area beneath the acromion, pain is relieved.

Diagnosis

Radiological examination occasionally shows the presence of calcification in the supraspinatus tendon.

Management

Rest and non-steroidal analgesics are the first line of management. If symptoms are very severe or persistent local infiltration of hydrocortisone and local anaesthetic into the subacromial bursa produces dramatic relief (Fig. 62).

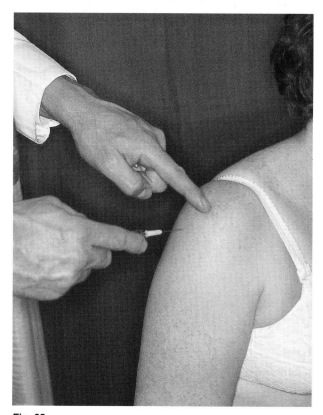

Fig. 62
The subacromial bursa can be injected from the lateral side as shown or anteriorly. The needle is passed under the acromion into the bursa and not into the rotator cuff itself.

Complications

- intratendonous injection with steroids may cause a tear in the rotator cuff.

Subacromial impingement

In older patients (40–60 years) there is chronic thickening of the rotator cuff from repeated 'wear and tear'. Associated with this may be arthritic degeneration of the acromioclavicular joint with osteophytes causing further impingement on the rotator cuff.

Clinical features

Patients present with similar symptoms and signs to those with supraspinatus tendonitis, but:

- Listen — there is a long history of repeated episodes of shoulder pain. Reaching upwards with the arm exacerbates the pain
- Look — patients tend to shrug the shoulder rather than abduct it
- Feel — there is tenderness over the rotator cuff
- Move — a painful arc of movement can be demonstrated as for acute supraspinatus tendonitis.

Management

This chronic impingement of a thickened rotator cuff in a narrowed subacromial space will not respond to anti-inflammatory agents and requires more space to be made by subacromial decompression of the rotator cuff by acromioclavicular joint incision and acromioplasty.

Complications

- rotator cuff tear.

Rotator cuff tear

Rotator cuff tears may be acute or degenerative, full thickness or partial thickness. Severe injuries to the shoulder in a young person produce an acute tear but in an old person a trivial injury may be sufficient to produce an acute tear in a degenerative rotator cuff.

Clinical features

There is pain on attempting to move the shoulder. In full thickness tears active movement is impossible. Initiation of abduction, particularly, is absent, but further abduction is possible by the action of deltoid. In partial thickness tears movement is possible but there is pain and weakness.

Diagnosis

An arthrogram (Fig. 63) or MRI scan will show the defect on the rotator cuff.

Management

In the young person, an acute rotator cuff tear can be treated by surgical repair. In the elderly, degenerative changes make repair unsuccessful, but a course of heat

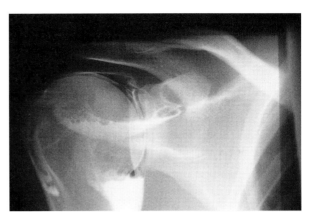

Fig. 63
Arthrogram of the shoulder showing a partial thickness tear of the rotator cuff.

treatment until symptoms settle followed by strengthening exercises over a full range of movement will produce an acceptable result.

Complications

- frozen shoulder (adhesive capsulitis) — disuse of the shoulder for whatever reason results in shrinking of the capsule and loss of movement in all directions.

Sporting shoulder injuries

Dislocations and fractures of the shoulder can occur particularly in those involved in sports.

Dislocations can be:

- anterior
- posterior
- inferior (luxatio erecta)
- associated with a fracture
- recurrent.

Anterior dislocation

This injury occurs with an abduction and extension force on the shoulder (Fig. 64). It is associated with falls and with sports.

Clinical features

- Listen — there is a history of a fall or a twisting injury of the shoulder
- Look — the affected shoulder appears flatter than normal on the lateral aspect. The tip of the acromion is prominent and is in line with the lateral epicondyle of the elbow giving a 'squared off' appearance to the shoulder on the affected side
- Feel — the humeral head may be palpable anteriorly. Loss of sensation on the 'badge patch' area must be sought, as if present it denotes damage to the axillary nerve at the humeral neck.
- Move — normal shoulder movements are impossible.

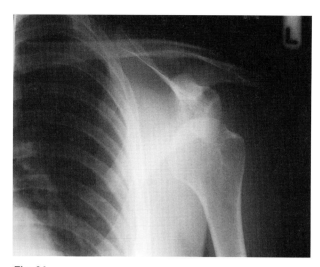

Fig. 64
Anterior dislocation of the shoulder.

Diagnosis

The diagnosis is usually obvious clinically but a radiograph should be taken to exclude an associated fracture. Radiographs can sometimes be difficult to interpret. Posterior dislocations are notorious for being overlooked as the humerus appears to be in joint. Close inspection, however, shows the characteristic 'light bulb' shape of the humeral heads as the tuberosities are not seen in their usual position.

Management

Occasionally, the shoulder may reduce spontaneously or by the 'hanging arm' technique in which the patient lies prone allowing the affected arm to hang vertically over the side of the couch. More usually, however, reduction under anaesthesia is required. Kochner's manoeuvre is commonly used, in which the arm is externally rotated and abducted, traction is applied with the help of a colleague's hand in the axilla and the arm is then swung into internal rotation and adduction across the patient's chest to be nursed there in a broad arm sling for 3–4 weeks while the anterior capsule heals.

Complications

- axillary nerve damage: this may occur during the injury or during the manipulation; the integrity of the nerve must always be checked for prior to attempting reduction. Absence of sensation over the point of the acromion suggests the nerve is damaged and, if it is, there will be resulting paralysis in the deltoid
- associated humeral fracture
- arterial damage: the axillary artery may be damaged
- stiffness known as 'frozen shoulder'
- irreducible dislocation: this is present if the humeral head button-holes through the rotator cuff; this happens only rarely but requires open reduction
- recurrent dislocation occurs if postoperative splintage is inadequate allowing resultant laxity of the soft tissues to develop.

Posterior dislocation

This condition is unusual but easily missed. Ligamentous laxity gives some patients the ability to voluntarily dislocate the shoulder posteriorly.

Diagnosis

The radiograph shows the characteristic 'light bulb' shape of the humeral head.

Management

Manipulation under anaesthesia followed by 3 weeks' immobilisation and subsequent physiotherapy.

Recurrent dislocation

Recurrent anterior dislocation occurs with extension and external rotation movements usually without any further trauma. Some patients report their shoulder dislocating while simply turning over in bed.

Diagnosis

Radiological examination shows flattening of part of the humeral head; the Hill–Sach's lesion. Elevation of the anterior glenoid rim and subscapularis muscle (the Bankart lesion) may be demonstrated by arthrography or MRI.

Management

Recurrent dislocation requires stabilisation of the shoulder by reefing the subscapular tendon (Putti–Platt operation), repairing the Bankart lesion or providing a dynamic anterior support by the transfer of the conjoint tendon through the subscapularis.

Fractured clavicle

This common injury is often associated with sports but can occur with any fall on the outstretched hand.

Clinical features

Pain and tenderness. The patient characteristically supports the weight of the arm with the opposite hand.

Diagnosis

The majority of injuries are in the middle third and occasionally there is overriding of the bone ends.

Management

The arm should be rested in a broad arm sling; sometimes a figure-of-eight bandage provides a comfortable brace for the shoulders.

Complications

- malunion
- damage to the subclavicular vessels
- non-union; this may be asymptomatic but, occasionally, requires open reduction, internal fixation and bone grafting

- deformity
- brachial plexus damage.

Acromioclavicular joint disruption

A fall on the point of the shoulder, classically during a rugby game, produces this injury.

Clinical features

The injury may be a sprain, a subluxation or a dislocation. The clavicle springs upward at the acromioclavicular joint producing a characteristic step on the shoulder.

Diagnosis

Radiographs comparing both shoulders while the patient carries weights in the hands are used to confirm a diagnosis and to differentiate between subluxations and dislocations.

Management

Conservative treatment is often all that is required, but occasionally fixation of the clavicle to the coracoid with a screw is carried out for those patients who require their shoulder for heavy work.

Complications

- pain
- weakness.

6.3 Rheumatoid arthritis

Rheumatoid arthritis (RA) is an inflammatory systemic disease of unknown aetiology, characterised by relapses and remissions, which may affect many joints simultaneously. An autoimmune inflammatory reaction in the synovium produces synovial hypertrophy and effusion. Eventually there is destruction of the articular cartilage, ligamentous laxity and erosion of the subchondral bone. These combine to result in mechanical derangement of the joint leading to subluxation and eventually permanent dislocation and deformity. The care of the rheumatoid patient progresses from medical treatment, often supervised by a rheumatologist, to combined care with an orthopaedic surgeon once surgical intervention is required.

Shoulder

Clinical features

- Listen — the shoulder is painful and limits function. It is difficult to comb the hair and reach to the perineum comfortably. Patients complain that they are unable to lie on the affected side
- Look — muscle wasting around the shoulder girdle
- Feel — joint swelling is not easy to detect. There may be tenderness at the acromioclavicular joint.

- Move — movements of the joint are painful and restricted, especially abduction and external rotation.

Diagnosis

Features of systemic disease may be present, such as elevation of the ESR and plasma viscosity. A positive RA latex may also be apparent but in approximately 30% of patients, this test is negative. Classically, radiographs of the wrists are used to look for early signs of rheumatoid authritis. Radiological examination of the affected joint shows:

- joint space narrowing
- marginal erosions
- osteopenia
- irregular joint surface
- eventually features of secondary osteoarthritis develop (Fig. 65).

Management

Medical management includes:

- drugs: therapy progresses from simple analgesics through steroids and NSAIDs to disease-modifying drugs such as penicillamine and gold; intra-articular injection of steroid and radioactive yttrium
- physiotherapy: preserves useful joint movement
- appliances to aid in the activities of daily living.

  Surgical management includes:

- arthroscopic synovectomy
- hemiarthroplasty of the humeral head is usually sufficient (Fig. 66)
- total shoulder replacement is required if the glenoid is severely eroded.

Complications

Complications of the disease:

- joint destruction

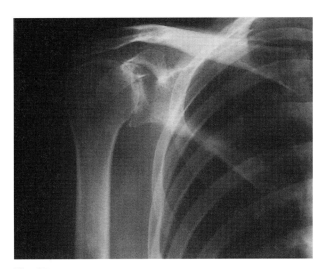

Fig. 65
Secondary osteoarthritis in the glenohumeral joint.

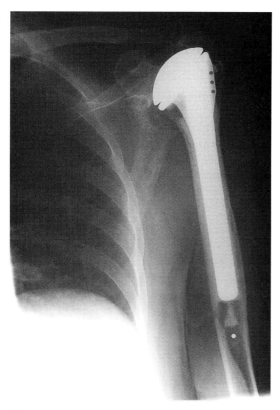

Fig. 66
Hemiarthroplasty of the shoulder for rheumatoid arthritis.

- dislocation
- rotator cuff degeneration.

  Complications of prosthetic replacement:

- infection
- loosening.

Elbow

Clinical features

Patients with rheumatoid arthritis involving the elbow may have involvement of the humero-ulnar, humero-radial, proximal radio-ulnar joint or a combination of any of them. In addition, there may be disease at the distal radio-ulnar joint.

- Listen — patients complain of pain and loss of function in the elbow. There may be difficulty with eating and washing and patients may complain of neck pain secondary to stretching forwards in an attempt to bring the mouth to the hand
- Look — swollen joint from synovial effusion; deformity of the bony contours due to subluxation
- Feel — crepitus and swelling
- Move — when the humero-ulnar joint is involved, the patient loses full flexion and extension and is unable to get the hand to the face. If the humero-radial or distal radio-ulnar joints are involved, there is loss of supination and pronation.

Diagnosis

Radiological examination shows features of RA (see above), but in addition excess bone resorption may be seen, which allows the olecranon to migrate proximally between the supracondylar ridges of the distal humerus.

Management

Conservative treatment includes drug therapy (p. 69) and splinting. Surgical management includes synovectomy, usually combined with radial head excision in cases of humero-radial joint involvement. Destruction of the humero-ulnar joint requires a total elbow replacement.

Complications
Complications of the disease include:

- progressive loss of function
- instability
- weakness.

Complications of surgery include:

- infection
- dislocation
- ulnar neuritis
- loosening of the prosthesis.

6.4 Elbow disorders

Elbow injuries associated with sport

Enthesopathy is the name given to discomfort at the site of origin of a muscle. It is caused by a tear in the muscle origin near the bone following repetitive activities involving lifting or stretching.

Tennis elbow/golfer's elbow

Clinical features
In tennis elbow there is pain over the lateral epicondyle of the elbow, which limits normal use. Local tenderness is found at the common extensor origin and symptoms can be exacerbated by stressing these muscles by forced palmar flexion of the wrist.

In golfer's elbow similar symptoms and signs are found on the medial side of the elbow at the common flexor origin. In this case, forced dorsiflexion of the wrist or resisted palmar flexion is painful.

Diagnosis
Radiological examination is unremarkable.

Management
Resting the elbow and avoiding particular activities may be all that is required. An above elbow splint can be used to enforce this. Infiltration of the common extensor or flexor origin with local anaesthetic and

steroid may produce some relief and can be repeated up to three times. Occasionally, surgical release is indicated, but the results are unpredictable.

Complications

Complications can arise from steroid injection:
- subcutaneous fat necrosis
- loss of skin pigmentation
- persisting symptoms.

Osteoarthritis

Arthritis in the elbow may be the result of heavy manual work or sports such as cricket.

Clinical features

There is pain, crepitus and loss of the full range of motion in the elbow.

Diagnosis

Radiological examination shows the features of osteoarthritis: joint space narrowing, osteophytes and subchondral sclerosis.

Management

Symptoms may be relieved by changing occupation and avoiding the use of the arm for strenuous activities. Occasionally, surgical debridement of osteophytes and release of joint capsule contractures can improve the range of movement but the results are often not maintained. In severe cases, total elbow replacement may be carried out, but the arm will not be suitable for heavy activities after this procedure.

Complications

- continuing pain
- loss of full range of movement.

Bursitis

Olecranon bursitis

This is either inflammatory or infective. Inflammatory bursitis is associated with rheumatoid arthritis, gout, other crystal arthropathies or direct trauma to the olecranon. Classically, this was described as resulting from pressure or friction on the olecranon, hence the original name of 'student's elbow'. Infective bursitis is usually due to staphylococcal infection.

Clinical features

There is a large fluctuant swelling at the olecranon associated with pain and redness. In infective bursitis, there is oedema, tenderness and spreading inflammation.

Diagnosis

Aspiration will help to identify the infecting organism and also to relieve the acute symptoms of inflammatory bursitis.

Management

A course of non-steroidal anti-inflammatory analgesics is sufficient for mild inflammatory disease. An appropriate antibiotic is necessary in addition for infected cases. Surgical excision of the bursa prevents recurrence.

Complications of surgery

- poor wound healing.
- sinus formation.

Self-assessment: questions

Multiple choice questions

1. In the 'painful arc syndrome':
   a. Calcification in the region of the supraspinatus tendon may be seen on X-ray radiographs
   b. The cause is a tear of the supraspinatus tendon
   c. Typically there is severe pain on initiating abduction
   d. Tenderness is generalised
   e. If untreated a 'frozen shoulder' often results

2. In rheumatoid arthritis:
   a. Radiographic features of osteoarthritis may be superimposed on those of rheumatoid arthritis
   b. Crepitus and pain may be produced by palpating the radial head while pronating/supinating the forearm
   c. Joint laxity allows a full range of shoulder movement to be retained in most patients
   d. Ulnar nerve dysfunction is rarely seen
   e. Synovectomy and radial head excision may relieve symptoms in the early stages of disease

Case histories

History 1

> A 50-year-old man falls heavily onto his right shoulder. He complains immediately of pain and loss of function. A radiograph taken in the Casualty Department shows no underlying fractures.

1. What diagnosis should be considered?
2. What would be looked for on physical examination?
3. How would the patient's condition be managed from now on?

History 2

> A 50-year-old accountant complains of an acute onset of severe pain in his dominant shoulder after a weekend spent painting his garden fence. Physical examination reveals well-localised acute tenderness just lateral and superior to the coracoid process.

1. What diagnosis should be suspected?
2. How should this patient be treated?

> Some years later he presents with a long history of continuing pain in his shoulder exacerbated by abduction.

3. What is the diagnosis this time?
4. How would management of the patient proceed at this stage?

Picture questions

Picture 1

Figure 67A shows a 30-year-old man who has suffered an injury to his left shoulder during a rugby match. The radiographic appearance of both acromioclavicular joints is seen in Figure 67B.

1. What abnormalities do you see?
2. How can this injury be managed?

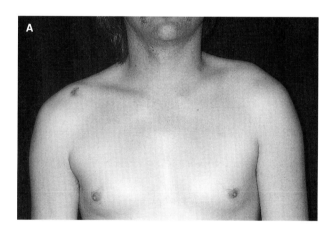

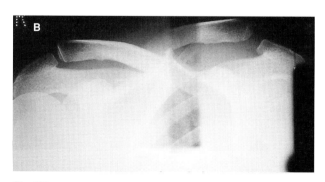

Fig. 67
A. 30-year-old man with an injury to his left shoulder. **B**. X-ray appearance of both acromioclavicular joints.

Picture 2

Figure 68 shows a radiograph of a rheumatoid elbow. List the radiographic features of rheumatoid arthritis to be seen.

Short notes

1. Write short notes on the presentation and clinical findings in tennis elbow.
2. List the information that should be given to a patient to enable them to give informed consent for the operation of total elbow replacement.

Viva questions

1. Demonstrate how the elbow can be examined to determine the range of movement.
2. A patient presents with a history of recurrent dislocation of the shoulder. What features would be expected on physical examination?

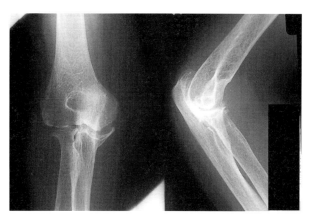

Fig. 68
Rheumatoid elbow.

Self-assessment: answers

Multiple choice answers

1. a. **True**. 'Painful arc syndrome' is caused by inflammation in the supraspinatus area of the rotator cuff, and calcification may occasionally be seen here on radiological examination.
   b. **False**. Tear of the supraspinatus part of the rotator cuff causes loss of ability to initiate abduction; although there may be pain in the shoulder, the painful arc is not present.
   c. **False**. The severe pain or painful arc syndrome is during the range from 30° to 60° as the inflamed swollen area of the rotator cuff passes beneath the acromion. There is no pain during the initiation of abduction.
   d. **False**. There is acute localised tenderness over the rotator cuff.
   e. **True**. If the patient is inhibited in the use of the shoulder because of pain then the capsule contracts and a frozen shoulder results.

2. a. **True**. Once the joint is destroyed by rheumatoid arthritis, secondary osteoarthritis may develop.
   b. **True**. Crepitus from motion between the two joint surfaces and pain on movement are readily found at the radial head during supination and pronation.
   c. **False**. Usually the destruction of the joint and the long period of immobility resulting from the pain have resulted in a loss of full shoulder joint movement.
   d. **False**. Ulnar neuritis is often associated with rheumatoid disease involving the elbow or wrist.
   e. **True**. Excision arthroplasty of the radial head and synovectomy reduce the disease process and the painful movements of the elbow. Dramatic relief can be achieved.

Case history answers

History 1

1. A fall onto the shoulder in a man of this age may cause a tear in the rotator cuff.
2. On physical examination, the appearance of the shoulder is normal but there is tenderness anteriorly over the rotator cuff and loss of the ability to initiate adduction. It is possible for the patient to hold the arm in adduction once this is initiated passively as the function of deltoid is not impaired. The inhibitory effect of localised pain as a cause of loss of function can be eliminated by local infiltration of anaesthetic into the subacromial bursa. Persisting loss of ability to initiate abduction suggests a mechanical cause. The diagnosis can be confirmed by arthrography or MRI.
3. Large tears can be repaired surgically but partial tears or tears in more elderly patients are best treated conservatively.

History 2

1. The history and clinical findings suggest a diagnosis of acute supraspinatus tendinitis.
2. Although this condition can be relieved by oral non-steroidal anti-inflammatory analgesics and rest, dramatic relief can be achieved immediately by an injection of a long-acting anaesthetic and steroid into the subacromial bursa.
3. A long history of painful abduction in the shoulder in an older patient suggests a diagnosis of subacromial impingement. The swollen rotator cuff is squashed beneath the arch of the acromion during abduction.
4. This time symptoms are unrelieved by steroid infiltration. An acromioplasty is often helpful.

Picture answers

Picture 1

The radiograph shows an acromioclavicular dislocation. This injury is usually managed conservatively by resting the arm in a broad arm sling until symptoms settle. In occasional patients where a full range of strong movements are required at the shoulder for work or sports, then open reduction and internal fixation of the clavicle to the coracoid process is required.

Picture 2

The radiographic features of rheumatoid arthritis visible on this radiograph are:

- joint space narrowing
- marginal erosions
- irregular joint surface
- osteopenia.

Short notes answers

1. Tennis elbow presents with a history of pain over the lateral epicondyle of the elbow, which limits normal use. There may be a history of repetitive activities such as lifting or stretching. Physical examination shows well-localised tenderness in the common extensor origin exacerbated by resisted dorsiflexion of the wrist or by full palmar flexion.
2. Prior to a total elbow replacement, the patient must be made fully aware of the intraoperative and

postoperative complications that may occur and understand the limitations of use that a prosthetic elbow replacement will impose on their life-style.

Intraoperative complications include:

- ulnar nerve damage
- fracture of the supracondylar ridges
- malalignment of the prosthesis.

Postoperative complications include:

- wound dehiscence
- deep infection
- ulnar neuritis
- dislocation.

The total joint replacement gives satisfactory pain relief but there may be a loss of full extension or flexion at the elbow. The joint is not able to withstand heavy lifting activities or manual work.

Viva questions

1. Movements that take place at the elbow are flexion, extension, supination and pronation. With the patient's arms fully stretched forwards, the elbows are in full extension. The affected side can be compared with the normal side. The range of movement from full extension to full flexion can be measured and compared with the opposite side. Usually full extension is recorded as $0°$ and full flexion as $130°$. To determine pronation and supination, it is important that the patient's elbows are tucked into the waist to prevent any auxiliary movement from the shoulder. With the hand in a fist and the palm upwards, the range of movement from full supination to full pronation can be observed and compared with the opposite side. Full supination is usually recorded as $90°$, neutral (with the fist vertical) $0°$ and full pronation as approximately $80°$.

2. A patient with a history of recurrent dislocation of the shoulder may exhibit apprehension on abduction and external rotation of the joint. Manipulation of the shoulder with the patient relaxed shows anterior laxity when an attempt is made to subluxate the humoral head from the glenoid.

Hand and wrist disorders

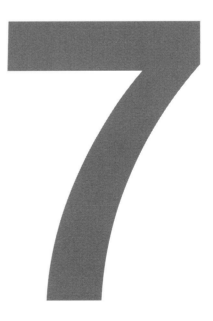

7.1 Clinical examination

Because of their exposed position in the body and their busy prehensile activity, the hand and wrist are vulnerable to injury in a variety of ways:

- cuts
- fractures/dislocations
- burns
- crushing
- infection.

Almost any combination of structures within the hand may be damaged in these ways so for any injured hand a checklist should be made of all the structures that could possibly be injured:

- skin
- tendons
- nerves
- vessels
- bone
- joints
- ligaments.

Much information can be gained from the careful examination of the hands not only for local pathology but also because the hands often manifest signs associated with remote or systemic diseases. Patients who have suffered a hand injury are very anxious and distressed about the effect this will have on normal hand function. Patients with infection in the hand will be in acute pain and resist the slightest attempts at examination. With so much information to be found from the hands, it is important to carefully follow the pattern of 'listen, look, feel, move'.

Listen. Several important questions must be asked, concerning:
- details of the injury
  — position the hand was in at the time
  — mechanism of injury
  — duration of contact of the hand with the injury force, e.g. crush from industrial rollers
- right- or left-handed
- occupation
- hobbies
- other activities involving precision use of the hand.

Look. Systematically look at each joint in the hand and wrist and remember to look at both palmar and dorsal surfaces. Do not forget to inspect the nails closely. In an exam, always describe what you are looking for and what you find to the examiner. Note any abnormal posture in the hand such as that associated with loss of function of a flexor or extensor tendon.

Feel. Palpate the surface of any swelling and determine whether it is in the skin or beneath the skin. See if the lesion moves in relation to the flexor tendon. Try to locate areas of tenderness very precisely with single digit palpation. Areas of altered sensation should be assessed by light touch and especially the moving two

point discrimination test. Patients should be able to feel the points of a pair of dividers or the ends of a paper clip two millimetres apart when they are being moved on the skin surface.

Move. Observe the passive and active range of movement of the joint. Remember that at the wrist ulnar and radial deviation can be measured and compared with the opposite side. Examine the fingers for the integrity of the flexor digitorum superficialis (FDS) and flexor digitorum profundus (FDP) tendons.

A careful history and examination should make it possible for you to predict exactly which structures have been injured.

Therapy
The worst complication of any injury to the hand is stiffness and contracture due to failure to prevent swelling or to encourage mobilisation. Sometimes, however, mobilisation is not possible and the hand must, therefore, be correctly splinted to avoid the development of contractures of the joints.

The correct position for splinting the hand is with the metacarpophalangeal joints in flexion and the proximal interphalangeal (PIP) joints in extension. In this position, the collateral ligaments of the joint are at their longest and, therefore, cannot contract. To aid this position, some dorsiflexion of the wrist is also used and is maintained by a plaster back slab. A bulky dressing on the palm of the hand is made with layers of fluffed gauze. If only the wrist is to be immobilised, it is important that the dressing does not impede motion of the more distal joints.

7.2 Fractures and dislocations

Phalanges

Clinical features
Fractures are caused by either twisting or angulating forces, may be stable or unstable and may be displaced or undisplaced (Fig. 69). The pull of the interossei on the proximal fragment causes it to flex, resulting in dorsal angulation at the fracture site as the extensors pull on the middle phalanx.

Management
Stable, undisplaced fractures can be splinted by the adjacent finger or a short metal splint, but interosseous wiring or crossed Kirschner wires may be necessary to stabilise an unstable fracture.

Dislocation of the interphalangeal joint

This common injury is usually easily reduced but is associated with either disruption of the collateral liga-

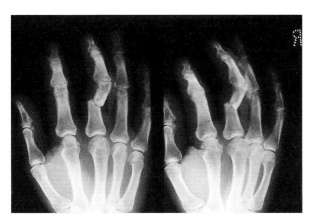

Fig. 69
Unstable transverse fracture of the proximal phalanx of the middle finger with posterior angulation and displacement.

ments or volar plate. There may be an associated avulsion fracture from the base of the adjacent phalanx.

Management
Reduction and splinting to the adjacent finger are usually sufficient but a large intra-articular fragment will require accurate internal fixation.

Complications

- stiffness caused by adhesion of extensor tendon at the fracture site
- malunion responsible for the rotated position of the finger, which becomes apparent with flexion
- flexion contraction due to scarring of the volar plate.

Metacarpals

Fifth metacarpal

The most commonly encountered fracture in the hand is a fracture of the neck of the fifth metacarpal (Boxer's fracture). The metacarpal head is usually rotated and angled towards the palm.

Management
Unless this angulation is more than 40° from the long axis of the metacarpal shaft, it can be ignored so long as rotation is controlled by strapping the small and ring fingers together. Angulation of more than 45° often requires reduction and stabilisation of the fracture by percutaneous Kirschner wires.

Complications

- extension lag
- stiff finger
- painful lump in the palm.

First metacarpal

Fractures of the first metacarpal may be:

- extra-articular: the fracture is usually transverse and above the level of the carpal joint

- intra-articular: the fracture is oblique, unstable, often displaced and involves part of the articular surface (Bennet's fracture; Fig. 70).

Clinical features
There is usually a history of a staving or punching injury. The base of the first metacarpal is prominent.

Management
Undisplaced fractures can be held in a plaster cast that is well moulded to the base of the metacarpal and extended to the tip of the thumb. Displaced fractures require reduction and fixation either by an interfragmentary screw or by stabilising the position of the first metacarpal relative to the second by transverse Kirschner wires from one to the other.

Complications

- malunion
- osteoarthritis.

Ulnar collateral ligament disruption at the MCP joint of the thumb

Acute abduction of the metacarpophalangeal joint of the thumb tears the ulnar collateral ligament and may avulse its origin on the base of the proximal phalanx. This injury commonly occurs in skiing or bike accidents. Chronic laxity of the ligament from repeated injury is called 'gamekeeper's thumb'.

Management
A Bennet's-type plaster is appropriate for partial tears but open reduction and intraosseous fixation are

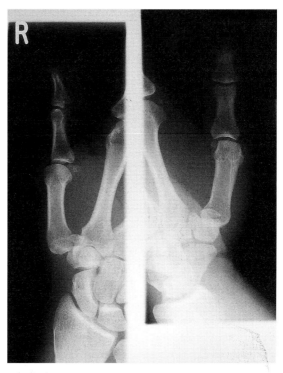

Fig. 70
Bennet's fracture of the first metacarpal.

required if the bony fragment is widely displaced or if the joint is very lax. In these cases the adductor aponeurosis will be interposed between the avulsed ligament and its insertion on the proximal phalanx.

Carpals

Scaphoid

Clinical features

Falls on the outstretched hand in young people may result in a fracture to the scaphoid bone.

- Listen — today the injury is often associated with sports, although at one time it was due to the kickback from a motor car starting handle.
- Look — swelling in the anatomical snuffbox
- Feel — there is localised tenderness in the anatomical snuffbox
- Move — pain is exacerbated by radial deviation of the wrist.

Diagnosis

Radiographs of the wrist in ulnar deviation show the scaphoid best and the type of fracture (stable, oblique, displaced) can be observed. Occult fractures may be more apparent if re-X-rayed a week later.

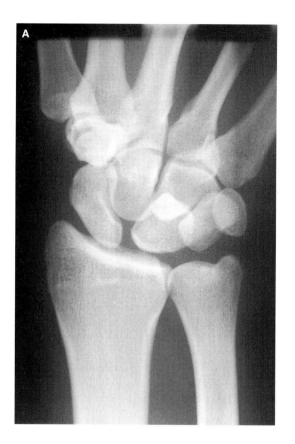

Management

Most scaphoid fractures can be treated conservatively in a plaster cast to immobilise the wrist while healing occurs. Unstable or displaced fractures require internal fixation with a screw to avoid progression to non-union.

Complications

- non-union
- avascular necrosis of the proximal fragment due to the retrograde blood supply to the scaphoid
- osteoarthritis and carpal collapse (SLAC wrist — scapholunate advanced collapse)
- persisting pain
- weak grip.

Dislocation of the lunate

A hyperextension injury of the wrist may dislocate the lunate anteriorly (Fig. 71) and produce acute symptoms of median nerve compression. Other more complex dislocations are associated with fractures of the scaphoid or capitate.

Management

Closed reduction may be possible followed by percutaneous wire stabilisation of the lunate, but often it is best to carry out an open reduction, repair the tear in the wrist capsule and decompress the carpal tunnel at the same time.

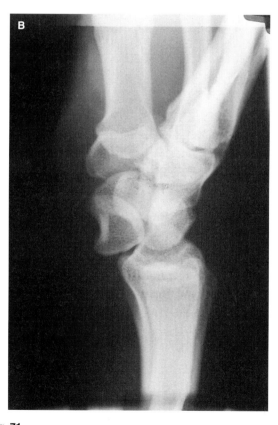

Fig. 71
Anterior–posterior (**A**) and lateral (**B**) radiographs of the wrist showing anterior dislocation of the lunate.

7.3 Injuries

Sharp injuries

Cuts to the hand frequently occur from falls onto broken glass or from cuts on a knife or metal edge. The skin wound often looks trivial so the depth of the wound and hence the damage to the underlying structures are frequently missed when patients attend the casualty department.

Clinical features
- **Listen** — An exact a description as possible of the mechanism of the injury should be elicited. The position the hand was in at the time of the accident is important. For example, if the fingers were cut gripping the blade while trying to resist a knife attack, then when straightened the position of the flexor tendon injury will be distal to the cut in the skin.
- **Look** — If a flexor or extensor tendon is divided the affected finger will be out of cadence with the other fingers, which normally fall into a resting position of partial flexion which increases from the index to the small finger. The site of the skin wound should be noted. Injuries on the palmar aspect of the proximal phalanx are likely to have divided both flexor tendons as they pass through the fibro-osseous tunnel in zone II (Fig. 72).
- **Feel** — Sensation on each side of the finger should be checked, although absence of touch sensation appears not to be registered immediately by patients despite division of a digital nerve. Eventually the denervated side of the finger feels very dry due to loss of sudomotor innervation.

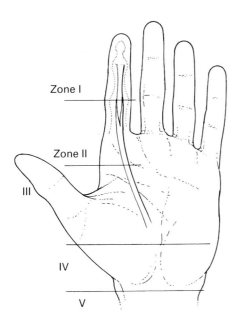

Fig. 72
Five zones of the hand showing the site of the fibro-osseous tunnel in zone II containing both flexor digitorum superficialis and flexor digitorum profundus in the fibrous flexor sheath.

- **Move** — Complete division of flexor digitorum superficialis causes loss of proximal interphalangeal joint flexion. If the adjacent fingers are held straight the injured finger is unable to flex at the peripheral interphalangeal joint. Complete division of flexor digitorum profundus causes loss of distal interphalangeal joint flexion when the finger is held straight at the proximal interphalangeal joint. Partial division is associated with painful weakness of these movements. If an extensor tendon is divided the finger hangs lower than its neighbours and cannot extend actively.

Diagnosis
The extent of injury to the underlying structures can be made clinically in most cases. If the injury was caused by a radio-opaque material a radiograph is useful to exclude any particles remaining in the wound.

Management
Tendons, nerves and vessels can all be repaired. The principles of surgery on the hand include the use of a bloodless field (produced by a tourniquet on the limb), magnification and appropriately fine instruments and suture material. The patient's hand should be rested on a table that is wide enough to allow the surgeon to rest his elbows on it while operating. In this way hand tremor is eliminated. If digital vessels and nerves are to be repaired the operating microscope should be used, but operating loupes magnifying between two and three times are sufficient for most procedures. Postoperative splinting to protect the repair together with exercises supervised by a hand therapist are required if a good result is to be achieved after these injuries.

Complications
- stiffness
- tendon adhesions
- cold intolerance
- numbness
- neuroma formation
- scar contracture.

Thermal injuries

Burns

Hands are also at risk from thermal injuries. As well as hot objects, other agents such as steam, hot liquids, flames, electricity and chemicals can cause burns.

Clinical features
Burns are classified (see Fig. 73) as:

- superficial (epidermal damage only) — epithelial cells remain in the hair follicles and sweat glands
- deep dermal (epidermis and some of the dermis are lost)
- full thickness (epidermis and dermis are totally destroyed).

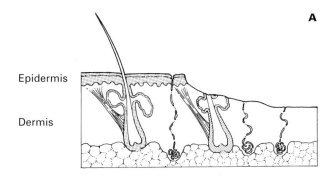

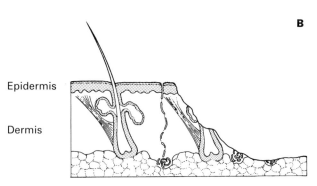

Fig. 73
A. In a superficial burn portions of the hair follicles and sweat glands with their associated epithelial linings remain to be the focus of epithelial regeneration. **B.** In a full thickness burn the epidermis and dermis are destroyed leaving no ability for epithelial regrowth to occur except from the wound edges.

Any burn of the hand is followed by swelling. This swelling interferes with movement of the hand and may cause permanent stiffness. It also interferes with healing of the skin. Larger and more severe burns are associated with more severe swelling.

Management
Minor burns are treated with small dressings that do not interfere with movement. More extensive burns are usually treated by placing the hand in a plastic bag and instructing the patient on elevation and mobilisation. Fingers must be put through a full range of movement to prevent stiffness and reduce the oedema, and thus promote healing. Deep dermal and full thickness burns will require excision and covering with a split thickness skin graft, which limits the risk of infection and the extent of scar contracture.

Cold injuries

Exposure of the fingers to extreme cold and damp may lead to frostbite.

Clinical features
There is discoloration, blistering and, ultimately, necrosis of the fingertips.

Management
The principles of treatment are the same as for burns. The hand should be elevated to prevent swelling and the patient

encouraged to exercise the digits. Eventually the areas of necrosis will demarcate and undergo dry gangrene. These will ultimately separate spontaneously, but amputation of necrotic areas will hasten the healing process.

Crush injuries

With crush injuries, it is important to know the nature of the crushing object. Often the injury involves industrial machinery. The size, weight, temperature or velocity of the equipment responsible may be of relevance. The length of time the hand was crushed must also be known.

Clinical features
A hand crushed between blunt objects or rollers may be swollen and bruised without definite injury to any of the internal structures. However, the skin may have been sheared (degloving injury) from the underlying structures and can be devascularised. Loss of capillary return helps to confirm this diagnosis.

7.4 Infection

Clinical features
Staphylococcal infection in the hand presents as a web space infection, paronychia or a tendon sheath infection. There is a collection of yellow pus, inability to move the affected finger and inflammation. Streptococcal infection is associated with a more insidious spreading infection, cellulitis, and ascending lymphangitis without the presence of pus at the original site.

Management
Pus under pressure must be released and the area washed out. Specimens are sent for bacteriological examination and intravenous antibiotics commenced. Flucloxacillin and fucidin are the 'best guess' for staphylococcal infections, but penicillin must be used if streptococcal infection is suspected.

Complications
- swelling
- contracture
- stiffness
- skin necrosis is seen in some cases of streptococcal infection.

7.5 Entrapment neuropathy

Pressure on a peripheral nerve in its fibro-osseous tunnel causes pressure on a localised section of the nerve that results in neuronal dysfunction causing characteristic features.

Carpal tunnel syndrome

Clinical features
Patients are usually female.
- **Listen** — The classical history is of pain at night in the radial three and a half digits, the distribution of the median nerve. There may be numbness, dysaesthesia and clumsiness.
- **Look** — There may be wasting of the muscles of the thenar eminence, especially abductor pollicis brevis, which is always innervated by the median nerve.
- **Feel** — There is altered or diminished sensation in the palmar aspect of the radial three and a half digits but not in the palm of the hand as the superficial branch of the median nerve supplying this area does not pass through the carpal tunnel.
- **Move** — There is weakness of abductor pollicis brevis. Tinel's sign, percussion over the median nerve at the carpal tunnel, exacerbates the symptoms, as does palmar flexion of the wrist (Phalen's sign).

Diagnosis
The diagnosis is usually made clinically but in equivocal cases nerve conduction studies are helpful, showing characteristic decreases in motor and sensory latency and of nerve conduction velocities at the wrist if the median nerve is significantly compressed.

Management
Conservative. Dorsiflexion splints to wear at night prevent wrist flexion during sleep and relieve symptoms. Local infiltration of a steroid into the carpal tunnel may be effective.

Surgical. Division of the flexor retinaculum achieves a dramatic improvement in symptoms. In cases of advanced thenar muscle wasting an opponensplasty to restore thumb opposition to the other digits can be achieved using flexor digitorum superficialis from the ring finger.

Cubital tunnel syndrome

Clinical features
- **Listen** — Pressure or traction on the ulnar nerve at the elbow causes pain and tingling in the distribution of the ulnar nerve.
- **Look** — There may be wasting of the hypothenar eminence and of the interossei. This is best seen in the first web space where the first dorsal interosseus is easy to see.
- **Feel** — There is altered sensation or numbness in both sides of the ulnar one and a half digits.
- **Move** — There is weakness of abductor digiti minimi and of abduction and adduction of all the fingers. Adductor pollicis is also weak resulting in a positive Froment's sign.

Diagnosis
Nerve conduction studies will confirm the diagnosis and localise the constricting lesion — usually a fibrous band between the two heads of flexor carpi ulnaris at the elbow.

Management
The ulnar nerve can be decompressed in the cubital tunnel by dividing the fibrous band. Traction on the nerve can be relieved by an anterior transposition, which relocates the nerve on the anterior side of the medial epicondyle.

7.6 Ganglia

The presence of a lump on the wrist or hand is a frequent complaint to present at the hand clinic. Ganglia are seen at the following sites:

- wrist: palm or dorsal aspects
- flexor tendon sheath
- distal interphalangeal joints.

The pathology causing a ganglion to develop is somewhat uncertain. Although ganglia communicate with a synovial lined cavity, such as a joint or the flexor tendon sheath, the fluid they contain is more gelatinous than pure synovial fluid. Although a pedicle can often be found connecting them to a joint (at the wrist this is usually the scapholunate joint), abnormal areas of joint capsule are found near the base where mucoid degeneration is taking place. Intraosseous and intratendinous ganglia are occasionally found.

Clinical features
Patients complain of a lump on the dorsum of the wrist or on the line of the flexor tendon sheath or on the dorsum of the distal interphalangeal joints. The lumps characteristically come and go but when present can be quite large and painful. Grip strength is impaired and the wrist may ache after prolonged use. Flexor tendon sheath ganglia are small and hard. They remain static while the finger flexes and extends and cause pain when gripping objects tightly. Ganglia at the distal interphalangeal (DIP) joints (usually referred to as mucous cysts) are unsightly. There is underlying osteoarthritis of the joint and the associated osteophytes are readily palpable.

Wrist ganglia are fixed to the underlying structures but not to the overlying skin. Their surface is smooth and they are often large and fluctuant but may be small and tense. On the palmar side, they are frequently in close conjunction to the radial artery.

Ganglia compressing the ulnar nerve as it passes through Guyon's canal, between the pisiform and the hook of the hamate, present with weakness of the muscles innervated by the ulnar nerve, altered sensation on the palmar aspect of the ulnar one and a half digits or with both motor and sensory abnormalities.

Diagnosis
Clinical examination is usually sufficient to make the diagnosis. A radiograph of the fingers will show the

underlying changes of osteoarthritis associated with a mucous cyst.

Management

Wrist ganglia were classically treated by dispersion as they were ruptured by being hit with a heavy object. Recurrence however is frequent after this procedure. Small ganglia can be managed by aspiration and injection of hydrocortisone, and this method is sometimes effective in flexor tendon sheath ganglia. The most reliable method is surgical excision. At the wrist ganglia must be carefully dissected from the radial artery and the stalk dissected back to the joint. Any abnormal areas of joint capsule must be removed at the same time. Flexor tendon sheath ganglia must be removed with a similar surrounding area of abnormal flexor tendon sheath. Careful dissection to ensure that the excision is complete will avoid recurrence. Mucous cysts require to be carefully dissected from the overlying skin. Osteophytes can be trimmed and the skin repaired. Sometimes a small rotation flap is necessary to close the defect.

Complications

- recurrence.

7.7 Dupuytren's contracture

Dupuytren's disease is a progressive contracture of the palmar fascia of the hand or foot of uncertain aetiology. Factors associated with the development of Dupuytren's contracture are:

- positive family history
- alcohol abuse
- diabetes
- anticonvulsant medication.

Clinical features

The disease usually affects the hands symmetrically and the ring and small fingers are usually the most severely involved. The condition may begin as a pit or a nodule in the palm before spreading distally as a cord to the digit and proximally to the base of the palm. Contracture of the cord produces flexion of the metacarpophalangeal and proximal interphalangeal joints. The presence of knuckle pads, involvement of the plantar fascia and a positive family history are associated with a poor prognosis and an increased recurrence rate after surgery.

Management

Surgical excision of the contracted cord is indicated if the metacarpophalangeal joint is flexed more than 40° or if there is any flexion of the proximal interphalangeal joint. Great care must be taken to protect the neurovascular bundles during the excision of the Dupuytren's tissue, which often winds round them

producing a spiral cord. Postoperative extension exercise and splintage are required to keep the finger straight.

Patients with recurrence often require multiple operations. Full thickness skin grafts are sometimes helpful to achieve healthy skin cover, but after several operations amputation of the affected digit may be necessary.

Complications

- recurrence in the same area after surgery
- extension to other parts of the hand
- maceration if left untreated
- cold intolerance ⎫ if the neurovascular bundles
- numbness ⎭ have been damaged.

7.8 Arthritis

Rheumatoid arthritis

The wrist and hand are common sites to be affected by rheumatoid arthritis.

Clinical features

Movements are restricted and painful.

- **Listen** — Painful joints cause difficulty with tasks of everyday life.
- **Look** — Swollen joints due to synovial hypertrophy and effusion are present. Muscle wasting may be seen in later stages. Characteristic deformities in the hand occur when the joints have become lax. They include radical deviation of the carpus and metacarpals, ulnar deviation of the phalanges, Z-shaped thumb, and boutonnière and swan neck deformities of the fingers (Fig. 74).
- **Feel** — Synovial effusion and hypertrophy may be felt over the metacarpophalangeal joints.
- **Move** — Joints may be immobile or very lax, allowing movement in any direction. If tendon ruptures have occurred then individual fingers will be floppy.

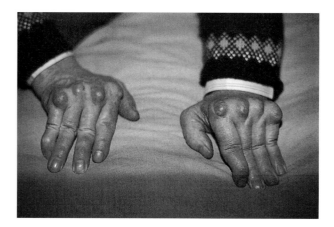

Fig. 74
Rheumatoid hand showing dislocation of the metacarpophalangeal joints and swan neck deformity of the fingers.

Diagnosis

Radiological features of rheumatoid arthritis are:

- osteopenia
- joint space narrowing
- marginal erosions
- joint subluxation and dislocation

and in later stages

- confluent, spontaneous arthrodesis of the carpus.

Management

Conservative
- splints
- analgesics, nonsteroidals and disease-modifying agents
- intra-articular steroids.

Surgical

- arthroplasty — replacement of the metacarpophalangeal joints and wrist
- arthrodesis — for stabilisation of the interphalangeal joints
- excision arthroplasty — excision of the distal ulna allows pain-free supination and pronation, and prevents further extenson tendon ruptures.

Complications

- progressive deformity
- loss of function
- loss of independence.

Osteoarthritis

In the hand, primary osteoarthritis is commonly seen in females over the age of 60 years. The sites affected are:

- distal interphalangeal joints
- carpometacarpal joint of the thumb
- triscaphie joint (between the scaphoid, trapezium and trapezoid)
- the proximal interphalangeal joint is rarely affected.

Secondary osteoarthritis can be precipitated by:

- intra-articular fractures
- septic arthritis
- carpal collapse — seen following scaphoid non-union

- Keinbock's disease (avascular necrosis of the lunate).

Clinical features
- Listen — patients complain of pain, weak grip and loss of function
- Look — the affected joints are swollen and stiff. There is deformity caused by osteophyte formation and eventually loss of function. At the dorsal interphalangeal joint, mucous cyst formation is seen as an eccentric dorsal swelling.
- Feel — tenderness and swelling
- Move — movements are limited and painful. Crepitus may be present.

Diagnosis

Radiological examination shows features of osteoarthritis:

- joint space narrowing
- subchondral sclerosis
- cysts
- osteophyte formation
- collapse.

Management

Conservative

- analgesics, splint

Surgical

The following armamentarium should be considered:

- arthrodesis for the distal interphalangeal joint and triscaphie joint
- interposition arthroplasty for the carpometacarpal joint of the thumb
- excision arthroplasty for the carpometacarpal joint of the thumb
- joint replacement for the interphalangeal joint of the middle or ring fingers.

Complications

- adduction deformity of first metacarpal following subluxation of arthritic first carpometacarpal joint
- first web space contracture
- weak pinch grip
- chronic pain.

Self-assessment: questions

Multiple choice questions

1. Carpal tunnel syndrome may be the consequence of:
   a. Pregnancy
   b. Dislocated lunate
   c. Fractured scaphoid
   d. Rheumatoid arthritis
   e. Fractured radial head

2. The radial nerve supplies:
   a. The extensors of the wrist
   b. The radial flexors of the wrist
   c. Abductor pollicis brevis
   d. Extensor pollicis longus
   e. Sensation to the tip of the thumb

3. In the hand:
   a. Boutonnière deformity results from rupture of the flexor digitorum tendon
   b. 'Trigger finger' may be caused by tightness of the flexor tendon sheath
   c. 'Mallet finger' is a flexion deformity of the proximal interphalangeal joint associated with trauma
   d. A functioning first dorsal interosseous muscle indicates intact motor function of the ulnar nerve
   e. Stenosing tenosynovitis (de Quervain's) affects the extensor pollicis longus tendon

Case histories

History 1

> A 60-year-old lady complains of pain in the radial side of her wrist when knitting. Osteoarthritis of the basal joint of her thumb is suspected.

1. What findings would be expected on examination?
2. What other features may be present that would suggest that the lady may have familial osteoarthritis?
3. Discuss the various management options appropriate for this condition.

History 2

> A 40-year-old female complains of pain in her fingers that wakes her at night. Further questioning reveals that it is the radial three and a half digits that are involved. Carpal tunnel syndrome is suspected.

1. What other questions would it be appropriate to ask?
2. What would you expect to find on clinical examination?
3. How could the severity of the condition be measured and quantified?

Picture question

Figure 75 shows a hand following a knife cut on the palmar side of the middle finger in zone I.
1. What structures do you think may be damaged in the finger?
2. How should the injury be managed?

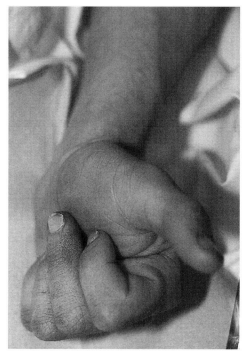

Fig. 75
Injury to the palmar aspect of the middle finger in zone I.

Short notes

Discuss the cause of the sudden loss of ability to extend the ring and small fingers in a rheumatoid hand. How can this disability be managed?

Viva questions

1. How should a patient with infective tenosynovitis be managed?
2. Demonstrate the examination of the hand required to assess the integrity of the flexor digitorum superficialis (FDS) and profundus (FDP).
3. How would you manage a division of flexor digitorum profundus in zone II?

Self-assessment: answers

Multiple choice answers

1. a. **True.** Fluid retention during pregnancy may cause carpal tunnel syndrome, which resolves when the baby is delivered.
   b. **True.** Anterior dislocation of the lunate causes direct compression of the median nerve.
   c. **False.**
   d. **True.** Synovial hypertrophy within the carpal tunnel causes median nerve compression in rheumatoid arthritis.
   e. **False.** The radial head is at the elbow but fractures of the distal radius may cause bleeding into the carpal tunnel and median nerve compression.

2. a. **True.**
   b. **False.** Flexor carpi radialis is supplied by the median nerve.
   c. **False.** Abductor pollicis brevis is supplied by the median nerve.
   d. **True.**
   e. **False.** Sensation at the tip of the thumb is supplied by the median nerve.

3. a. **False.** The boutonnière deformity is caused by rupture of the central slip of the extensor tendon over the proximal interphalangeal joint.
   b. **True.** Constriction at the mouth of the flexor tendon sheath at the level of the first annular pulley produces local swelling of the tendon that prohibits its gliding into the mouth of the tendon sheath, producing a snapping movement called triggering.
   c. **False.** 'Mallet finger' is used to describe the inability to extend the distal interphalangeal joint following traumatic rupture of the extensor tendon or avulsion of a bony fragment from the base of the terminal phalanx.
   d. **True.** The first dorsal interosseous muscle is supplied by the ulnar nerve and its muscle belly can be readily seen in the first web space.
   e. **False.** De Quervain's tenosynovitis refers to symptoms related to the first dorsal compartment containing the tendons of abductor pollicis longus and extensor pollicis brevis.

Case history answers

History 1

1. In osteoarthritis of the basal joint of the thumb, there is pain on moving the thumb at the carpometacarpal joint. The joint is often subluxated and attempting to reduce it causes pain. The first web space is often contracted.

2. Familial primary osteoarthritis often presents with Heberden's nodes, which are osteophytes at the distal interphalangeal joints.
3. Painful osteoarthritis at the basal joint of the thumb can be treated by arthrodesis if the adjacent joints are not destroyed. If there is pantrapezial disease, then excision of the trapezium with insertion of a soft tissue spacer is indicated. Silastic spacers and prostheses to resurface the joint have also been used.

History 2

1. Patients with carpal tunnel syndrome may also complain of tingling, numbness or dysaesthesia in the radial three and a half digits.
2. Clinical examination reveals numbness, weakness of abductor pollicis brevis and increased two point discrimination. Tinel's test is positive at the wrist and Phalen's test may also be positive.
3. Nerve conduction studies are used to assess the severity of the condition.

Picture answer

1. A cut on the hand at the site shown may have divided the underlying flexor tendons and neurovascular bundles. In zone I only flexor digitorum profundus is present and loss of function of this tendon is demonstrated by loss of flexion of the distal interphalangeal joint.
2. Initial management involves cleaning and exploring the wound under appropriate anaesthesia. The tendon can be repaired and a microneurorrhaphy carried out. If cold intolerance is to be avoided the digital vessels should be repaired too if they are divided. Postoperative splintage is required to protect the tendon repair by inhibiting full extension, and at the same time supervised flexion exercises are required to prevent adhesion formation and stiffness.

Short notes answer

In rheumatoid arthritis, the extensor tendons may rupture spontaneously at the wrist, especially under the extensor retinaculum where they are invaded by rheumatoid synovium. Attrition rupture can also occur at this site if the tendons rub on the exposed head of the ulna.

Treatment for rupture of extensor tendons in rheumatoid arthritis consists of suturing the ruptured tendon to an intact neighbour. Tendons that have been cut can be sutured together directly, but tendons that have spontaneously ruptured or worn through cannot because their ends are frayed and thin.

Viva answers

1. Infective tenosynovitis must be managed by an intensive course of an appropriate antibiotic. Specimens of pus are sent for bacteriological examination. If staphylococcus is suspected, then flucloxacillin is used, but if a streptococcal infection is present then benzyl penicillin is the antibiotic of choice. Drainage of the flexor tendon sheath with irrigation must be carried out, the hand elevated and active and passive finger flexion encouraged to prevent the development of adhesions.

2. The integrity of flexor digitorum superficialis is assessed by examining the hand with the fingers fully extended. Allowing the affected finger to flex at the proximal interphalangeal joint demonstrates its action. With all the fingers held in full extension, the terminal phalanges are allowed to flex together. This action indicates the integrity of the flexor digitorum profundus.

3. The division of the flexor digitorum profundus in zone II is treated by opening the flexor tendon sheath and by repair using a core stitch and a running circumferential inverting suture. After surgery, hyperextension of the wrist and fingers must be prevented by a splint and intermittent passive motion instituted to prevent adhesion formation.

Hip disorders

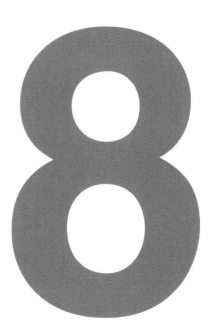

8.1 **Clinical examination**

In addition to the usual 'listen, look, feel, move', examination of the hip includes observation of the patient walking, standing and lying.

Walking. Observe for short leg gait, antalgic gait or Trendelenburg gait.

Standing. Observe the pelvic tilt while standing on each leg in turn. A positive Trendelenburg sign is present when the patient's pelvis dips to the opposite side while weight-bearing on the affected leg (Fig. 76).

Lying. With the patient lying supine, movements of the hip joint can be measured. These include flexion and extension, abduction and adduction and internal and external rotation. Care must be taken to ensure that the pelvis does not move during these manoeuvres, and this can best be achieved by stabilising the pelvis with one hand while manipulating the leg with the other. True and apparent leg lengths should be measured. True leg length is measured with the hips in the identical degree of adduction, measuring from the anterior superior iliac spine to the medial malleolus. Apparent leg length is measured with the legs parallel to each other measuring from the umbilicus to the medial malleolus. Finally Thomas's test, which unmasks a fixed flexion deformity of the hip, should be performed by flexing the unaffected hip up to the chest wall and observing whether the leg on the affected side rises off the couch during this manoeuvre.

8.2 **Arthritis**

Osteoarthritis of the hip is a common condition, affecting patients usually in their sixties and seventies. Primary osteoarthritis occurs idiopathically but is sometimes associated with a positive family history.

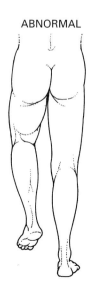 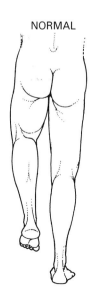

ABNORMAL   NORMAL

Fig. 76
Positive Trendelenburg test.

Secondary osteoarthritis can develop following previous insults to the joint from:

- trauma
- infection
- avascular necrosis
- Perthes' disease.

The sequence of pathological changes in the articular cartilage begins with fibrillation and cleft formation of the articular surface secondary to breaks in the normal arcades of collagen fibres. Clefts develop in the articular cartilage and the intracellular enzymes released cause synovial irritation. The resulting inflammation leads to contracture of the capsule. Eventually, articular cartilage is destroyed and subchondral bone becomes exposed. Cysts may develop in the subchondral bone and contribute to the femoral head collapse.

Clinical features

The main clinical features are:
- pain
- stiffness
- loss of function.

Listen. The severity of pain should be graded to assess the severity of the condition. A useful scale is one ranging from pain that is present with vigorous activity, through pain that is present with weight-bearing, to pain that is present at rest and, ultimately, pain that prevents sleep. Pain is often referred to the groin and thigh and sometimes the misleading symptom of pain at the knee is the presenting feature of hip disease.

Look. Examination of the patient walking may show an antalgic gait, a Trendelenburg gait or a short-leg gait (see Fig. 76).

Feel. Because the hip joint is deeply situated little can be felt by palpation, but tenderness may be elicited by percussion over the greater trochanter.

Move. There is limited range of movement and in particular there are flexion and abduction contractures with loss of internal rotation. Flexion contractures can be unmasked by Thomas's test, which corrects the secondary hyperlordosis of the lumbar spine.

Diagnosis

Radiological examination shows joint space narrowing, subchondral sclerosis, osteophyte formation and subchondral cysts (Fig. 77).

Management

General. Some simple advice may be helpful. The patient may be able to live within the limits of their discomfort without further treatment. Weight reduction may help. The use of a walking stick in the opposite hand decreases the load crossing the painful hip. If there is leg length inequality, a shoe raise is used to

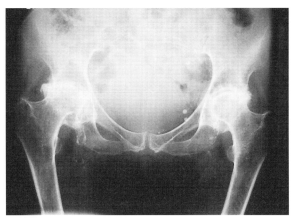

Fig. 77
Bilateral osteoarthritis of the hips with loss of the joint space, subchondral sclerosis, osteophytes and subchondral cysts. Very extensive femoral head collapse.

correct the gait and so relieve secondary back pain. Physiotherapy has a role in keeping other joints mobile.

Medical management. Analgesics and non-steroidal anti-inflammatory drugs are useful, although there is a risk of gastrointestinal haemorrhage with these.

Surgical management. The mainstay of surgical management has become a total joint replacement, but this is not always the most appropriate option. Other procedures to be considered include:

- osteotomy
- arthrodesis
- arthroplasty.

Osteotomy

Cutting the femur in the area of the trochanters and displacing the fragments can be used to rotate the head and realign the joint (Fig. 78). This has the effect of altering the weight-bearing surface, reducing the load across the hip joint and achieving vascular decompression of the bone. Symptoms may be relieved and joint function improved. Osteotomy is appropriate for a young patient with only an isolated point of arthritis in the joint.

Arthrodesis

Fusion of the hip joint with a bone graft achieves pain relief but at the expense of loss of movement. The knee, back and contralateral hip must have free painless movement to compensate for the arthrodesed joint. This debilitating operation may be considered in severe arthritis in a young patient.

Excision arthroplasty

If the affected joint is excised, the 'gap' fills with fibrous tissue. The leg is several centimetres shorter after this procedure but painless movement is possible. This is usually reserved as a revision operation following removal of an infected joint replacement.

Total joint replacement

A total joint replacement involves replacement of both

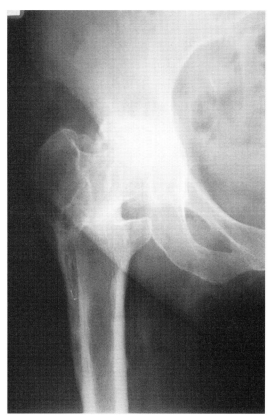

Fig. 78
Osteoarthritis of the hip which has previously been treated by an intertrochanteric displacement osteotomy.

the acetabular and femoral parts of the joint. An acetabular cup made of high-density polyethylene and a metal femoral component are used (Fig. 79). These are cemented into the bone with acrylic cement. Prophylactic antibiotics and precautions against deep venous thrombosis and pulmonary embolism are usually employed. Reliably good results can be achieved but there is a long-term risk of recurrence of hip pain if the implant becomes loose or infected. Revision surgery is then required. Patients should be prepared to limit their activities in an attempt to avoid the development of loosening and further surgery.

Complications of surgery

- chest infection
- urinary tract infection
- pressure sores
- deep vein thrombosis and pulmonary embolus.

Specific complications

- early
  — haematoma formation
  — wound dehiscence
  — wound infection
  — dislocation
- late
  — aseptic loosening
  — deep infection.

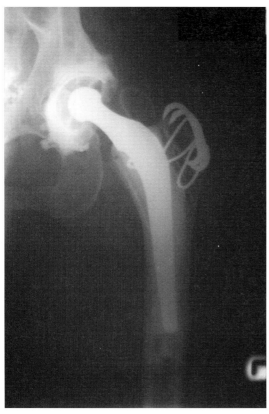

Fig. 79
Arthritis of the hip treated by a Charnley total hip replacement.

8.3 Hip injuries

Hip injuries in young people

Whereas fractures of the femoral neck are commonplace low-energy injuries in elderly women, a similar fracture in a young adult is uncommon but, when present, indicates the involvement of a high-energy injuring force. Fractures are, therefore, commonly comminuted and may extend into the upper third of the femur (subtrochanteric fractures) or involve the femoral head.

Clinical features

- pain
- excessive swelling of the hip and thigh
- the leg is externally rotated and shortened
- injuries to adjacent soft tissues
- injuries elsewhere.

Diagnosis

Plain radiographs will show the fracture fragments.

Management

High fractures of the femoral neck are stabilised by screw fixation, but subcutaneous fractures can be more difficult. Operative stabilisation with an intramedullary device such as the 'reconstruction nail' is used and allows early active movement and weight-bearing (Fig. 80).

Complications

- of the injury
  — shock
  — damage to adjacent soft tissues
- of surgery
  — wound infection
  — delayed union
  — non-union.

Dislocation

A high-energy injury is required to dislocate the hip. Involvement in a road traffic accident is a common history. Dislocations can be classified as:

- posterior dislocation
- anterior dislocation
- central dislocation.

Posterior dislocation

As the hip has dislocated posteriorly there may be an associated fracture of the posterior lip of the acetabulum or of the head of the femur itself.

Clinical features

- **Listen** — There is a history of a direct blow to the knee while seated, often from the car dashboard in a road traffic accident.

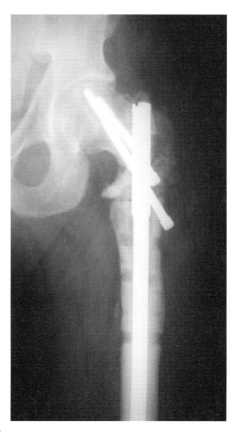

Fig. 80
Reconstruction nail used in the treatment of a subtrochanteric fracture previously treated unsuccessfully with a sliding nail plate.

- **Look** — The leg lies in a characteristic position of adduction and internal rotation and appears short. There is often flexion of the hip and knee. There may be a telltale injury over the knee.
- **Feel** — Sciatic nerve compression from the displaced femoral head causes altered sensation in the leg.
- **Move** — Hip movements are resisted, and with sciatic nerve compression there may be weakness of ankle movement.

Diagnosis

Plain radiographs show the dislocation and any major fractures of the acetabular margin, but small fractures, especially displaced fragments of a femoral head fracture, will be best seen by CT scan (Fig. 81).

Management

Urgent reduction of the dislocation is required as avascular necrosis of the femoral head will occur if stretching of the capsular vessels to the femoral head is prolonged. Open reduction may be required, especially if exploration of the sciatic nerve is thought to be necessary or if there is a posterior acetabular lip fragment requiring internal fixation. Small bone fragments within the joint must be removed, but a large fragment from the femoral head should be secured back in place with screws.

Complications

- sciatic nerve damage
- avascular necrosis
- secondary osteoarthritis.

Anterior dislocation

This injury is rare. The leg lies in external rotation, abduction and flexion. The dislocation can be reduced by manipulation under anaesthesia. Again, avascular necrosis is a complication.

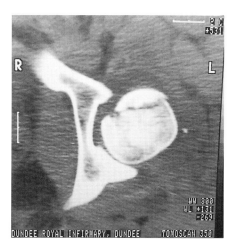

Fig. 81
CT scan of a reduced dislocation of the hip showing an associated fracture of the femoral head.

Central dislocation

High-energy injury is required to produce this dislocation, which is really a fracture of the floor of the acetabulum.

Diagnosis

A plain radiograph shows a comminuted fracture with central displacement of the femoral head into the pelvis (Fig. 82A). There are various degrees of displacement of the femoral head and multiple fragments of bone may be present, which can best be identified by a CT scan (Fig. 82B). This will assist in planning the stabilisation of the fracture by internal fixation.

Management

The hip can be reduced by manipulation under anaesthesia, although internal fixation of the fragments of the acetabular floor by contoured plates and screws is a preferable but more difficult approach requiring considerable expertise.

Complications

- secondary arthritis.

Fractured pelvis

Fractures of the pelvis can range from trivial to life-threatening.

Fractured pubic rami

A minor fall in an elderly patient is often the cause of a fracture of one or more pubic rami.

Clinical features

After a minor fall, the patient complains of discomfort around the hip and groin. Clinical examination reveals no evidence of fracture of the femoral neck or greater trochanter (which are other likely sites of injury) but there is localised tenderness at the pubic rami and maybe bruising and swelling here later.

Diagnosis

Plain radiographs will confirm the diagnosis. Both pubic rami on the same side are usually injured.

Management

The patient rests until the discomfort has settled and then gradual mobilisation begins over the following few days.

Complications

- none except those related to bed rest.

Acetabular fractures

Major trauma to the pelvis directed via the greater trochanter or along the axis of the femur fractures either the anterior or posterior columns of the acetabulum. These columns represent the strong bony margins of the pelvis which enclose the acetabulum.

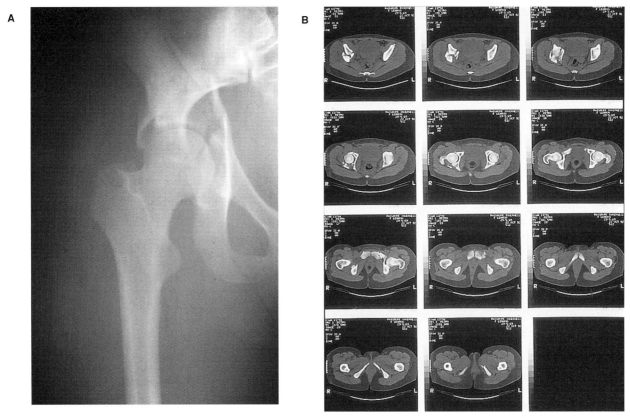

Fig. 82
A. Central dislocation of the hip with a comminuted fracture of the acetabulum. **B**. CT scan showing the position of the multiple fragments of an acetabular fracture.

Clinical features

There is localised tenderness and bruising around the pelvis with pain on stressing the pelvic ring. The patient may be profoundly shocked from extensive bleeding from the pelvic veins.

Diagnosis

X-rays at 45° will show the anterior and posterior columns more effectively than antero-posterior films. CT scan will show the details of the injury more precisely.

Management

Initial management involves the restoration of acute blood loss by intravenous fluids. In the younger patient, open reduction and internal fixation with malleable plates is required. This is commonly preceded by an arteriogramy and intravenous urogramy. Alternative treatment in an elderly or debilitated patient is traction until the fracture stabilises.

Complications

• acute blood loss
• other injuries to the axial skeleton
• damage to the bladder or ureter.

Fractures of the pelvic ring

With severe injuries, the pelvis may break:

• on either side of the midline
• in both its anterior and posterior parts.

In either of these mechanisms, a floating segment is produced.

Fractures on either side of the midline

Clinical features. A direct blow from the front may fracture all four pubic rami, creating a floating segment incorporating the fragments attached to the pubic symphysis, the bladder and the urethra (Fig. 83). There is a boggy swelling and bruising in the perineum. There may be extraperitoneal extravasation of urine, haematuria or blood at the urinary meatus.

Diagnosis. Plain radiographs show the fracture but the presence of urinary tract rupture must be sought by intravenous urethrograms.

Management. Initially, circulating volume must be restored as internal bleeding may be extensive. A single attempt is usually made to pass a urethral catheter, but if this fails suprapubic drainage must be commenced, usually by a urologist. Bladder and urethral repair may be required. Definitive open reduction and internal fixation can be attempted later.

Complications

• circulatory collapse
• bladder rupture
• urethral tear.

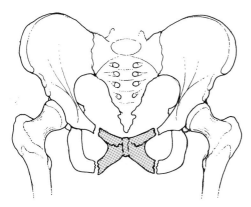

Fig. 83
Fracture of all four pubic rami creating a floating segment.

Fractures of both anterior and posterior sides

Clinical features. Disruption of the pelvic ring with anterior and posterior injuries creates a floating segment of one half of the pelvis. There may be fractures of two ipsilateral pubic rami together with a posterior fracture of the ilium or a separation of the sacroiliac joint. Stressing the pelvis produces pain. One half of the pelvis is obvious higher than the other creating a difference in leg length.

Diagnosis. X-rays show the extent of the disruption.

Management. The fragments can be brought down and stabilised by emergency external fixation which reduces bleeding from the iliac vessels and so restores haemodynamic stability. Definitive internal fixation can be carried out later.

Complications

- circulatory collapse
- sacral nerve root disruption.

8.4 Avascular necrosis

Avascular necrosis of the femoral head may be idiopathic but is also associated with alcohol abuse and deep sea diving. Sometimes it is secondary to infection or to intracapsular fractures or dislocations of the hip. The avascular bone becomes sclerotic, collapses and dies.

Clinical features
The hip joint is stiff and painful and the patient walks with a limp.

Diagnosis
Radiological examination shows collapse and sclerosis of the avascular femoral head with osteoporosis of the surrounding bone.

Management
Treatment of the early painful phase of avascular sclerosis is difficult. Osteotomy and core excision of the femoral neck and head have been used in an attempt to stimulate revascularisation. An operation to insert a vascularised iliac crest bone graft has also been used in an attempt to bring a new external blood supply to the hip. Once osteoarthritic changes have developed total joint replacement is necessary.

Complications

- secondary osteoarthritis.

Self-assessment: questions

Multiple choice questions

1. Recognised complications of a posterior dislocation of the hip are:
   a. Anterior acetabular rim fracture
   b. Avascular necrosis of the femoral head
   c. Femoral nerve injury
   d. Chondromalacia of the femoral head
   e. Sciatic nerve injury

2. Emergency management of the patient with a high-velocity pelvic ring fracture includes:
   a. Longitudinal traction to the affected limb
   b. Passing a urethral catheter
   c. Institution of intravenous infusion with large volumes of crystalloids
   d. Exclusion of other life-threatening injuries
   e. External fixation of the pelvic fractures

3. Which of the following radiographic features are commonly seen in osteoarthritis:
   a. Subchondral cysts
   b. Marginal erosions at the joint
   c. Osteophytes
   d. Looser's zones
   e. Heterotropic calcification

Case history

A 50-year-old labourer presents with a 12-month history of increasing pain in the right hip that often disturbs him at night and on days off.

1. How could the severity of his pain be graded?
2. What examination should be done?
3. What general advice should the patient be given?
4. Discuss which surgical method of treatment you would suggest and why this would be appropriate for this patient.

Picture question

Figure 84 shows the pelvis of a 45-year-old barmaid.
1. What radiographic features can be seen?
2. What is the diagnosis?
3. Discuss the treatment options available.

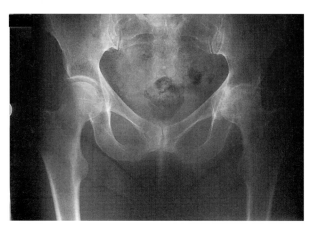

Fig. 84

Short notes

1. List the complications of which the patient should be aware before giving informed consent to a total hip replacement under general anaesthesia.
2. List the surgical methods of treating arthritis and illustrate each of them with reference to a particular joint.

Viva questions

1. What would be the duties of a preregistration house officer attending a patient the day after a total hip replacement?
2. What are the advantages and disadvantages of open reduction and internal fixation of a hip fracture in the young adult?

Self-assessment: answers

Multiple choice answers

1. a. **False.** In posterior dislocation of the hip, it is the posterior margin of the acetabulum which may be fractured.
   b. **True.** Damage to the vessels supplying the femoral head will result in avascular necrosis, especially if the dislocation is not urgently reduced.
   c. **False.** The femoral nerve lies anteriorly and is not in jeopardy.
   d. **True.** Even a moderate degree of ischaemia to the femoral head will result in death of the articular cartilage.
   e. **True.** The dislocated head may directly compress the sciatic nerve, which lies posteriorly.

2. a. **False.** Disruption of the pelvic ring requires urgent reduction to compress the pelvis. Longitudinal traction on the leg would not achieve this.
   b. **True.** Urethral damage is suspected in the presence of perineal bruising, scrotal haematoma or blood at the urethral meatus. The integrity of the urethra can be verified by passing a catheter.
   c. **True.** Large volumes of blood are lost from pelvic fractures and rapid intravenous restoration of the circulating volume is mandatory.
   d. **True.** The presence of one high-velocity injury should alert staff to the possibility of other severe injuries to the chest or abdomen.
   e. **True.** An external fixator placed between the iliac spines will reduce a displaced fracture of the pelvic ring and decrease haemorrhage.

3. a. **True.**
   b. **False.** These are associated with rheumatoid arthritis.
   c. **True.**
   d. **False.** These are associated with osteomalacia.
   e. **False.** This can be the sequelae of an intramuscular haematoma.

Case history answer

1. Severity of pain can be graded according to how much it interferes with activities and rest.
2. Examination of the patient would include a complete examination of the hips and also of the back, knees and general health of the patient.
3. General advice to this patient might include discussion about change of job, altering his pattern of work and weight reduction. The use of simple analgesics or non-steroidal anti-inflammatory drugs could be discussed.

4. The choice of surgical management of this patient is not easy. A total joint replacement, although indicated from his degree of pain and disability, would not withstand the forces put on it by his employment. An osteotomy incorporating decompression and rotation of the femoral head may give some relief by vascular decompression of the bone and redistribution of load across the joint. Subsequent total joint replacement could be carried out later.

Picture answer

1. Sclerosis of the femoral head.
2. Avascular necrosis.
3. Osteotomy, core excision. Ultimately a total hip replacement would be required.

Short notes answers

1. General complications of hip surgery under general anaesthesia include:
   - aspiration of gastric contents
   - chest infection
   - deep venous thrombosis and pulmonary embolism.

   Specific complications of a total hip replacement include:

   - wound infection
   - dislocation
   - nerve and vessel damage.

   Long-term complications include:

   - persisting pain and stiffness with continued limitation of activities
   - loosening of the prosthesis
   - the possibility of revision surgery for later infection.

2. The following surgical methods of treating arthritis are available:
   Osteotomy. A lateral closing wedge osteotomy of the upper tibia is used to treat medial compartment arthritis in the knee.
   Arthrodesis. Hallux rigidus can be treated by arthrodesis of the first metatarsophalangeal joint in the appropriate degree of dorsiflexion.
   Excision arthroplasty. Arthritis around the radial head can be treated by excision arthroplasty of the radial head without the use of a prosthetic spacer.
   Interposition arthroplasty. Arthritis of the basal joint of the thumb can be treated by interposition arthroplasty with a silastic spacer or soft tissue 'anchovy'.

Bipolar arthroplasty. Arthritis of the hip in selected patients is treated with a bipolar arthroplasty without formally resurfacing the acetabulum.

Total joint replacement. This is the final method of treating arthritis and involves replacing both surfaces of the joint with components of metal and high-density polyethylene.

Viva answers

1. The house officer would be responsible for:
   - pain relief
   - prophylactic measures to prevent postoperative infection and deep venous thrombosis
   - fluid balance
   - Monitoring of temperature, blood pressure and heart rate
   - checking the radiographs of the prosthesis.

2. The advantages of using open reduction and internal fixation of a hip fracture in a young adult are the restoration of normal anatomy, the institution of early mobilisation of the adjacent joints and the early discharge of the patient from hospital and eventual rapid return to work.

   The disadvantages are the risk of introducing infection, creating a stress riser at the end of the rodded bone and the later inconvenience of having the device taken out when the fracture has healed.

Knee disorders

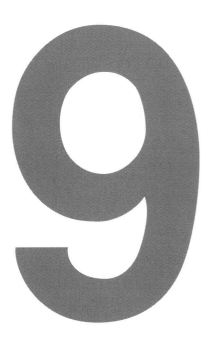

9.1 The clinical examination

The knee joint is very superficial, so much of its structure can be observed and palpated. Examination can be very precise, and if done carefully will help you extensively in making a diagnosis. Being asked to examine the knee is a common question in undergraduate clinical examinations as patients with specific clinical findings are readily available. It is very important, therefore, that you are proficient at the examination technique involved. This, as always, includes 'listen, look, feel and move'. Do not forget to observe the patient walking and standing as well as lying down.

- **Listen.** Key features in the history include:
  — mechanism of injury
  — pain
  — instability
  — swelling or locking.
- **Look:**
  — varus/valgus alignment
  — effusion in the suprapatellar pouch
  — scars from previous injury or surgery
  — do not forget to look behind the knee for a popliteal cyst.
- **Feel** — With the knee flexed to 90° the medial and lateral joint lines can be palpated. The origins and insertions of the medial and lateral collateral ligaments may be tender if they have been stretched or torn.
- **Move** — Carry out the anterior draw sign to check for anterior cruciate laxity. Observe for the presence of a posterior sag suggestive of posterior cruciate ligament rupture. Apply varus and valgus stresses to the partially flexed knee to check the integrity of the medial and lateral collateral ligaments. Observe the knee for evidence of locking (a block to full extension) and demonstrate that full flexion is possible.

9.2 The 'sportsman's knee'

Knee injuries are often caused by sporting activities.

Meniscus

Meniscal tears are the most common injury to the knee. They are caused by twisting injuries while weight-bearing on the affected leg. As seen in those involved in sport they are usually vertically orientated and may form part of a triad of injuries which includes damage to the medial collateral and anterior cruciate ligaments. In an older patient the meniscus becomes degenerate and minor twisting forces may be enough to cause meniscal tears which are usually orientated horizontally (Fig. 85).

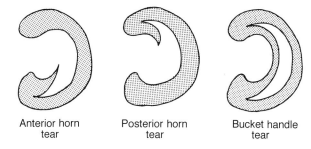

| Anterior horn tear | Posterior horn tear | Bucket handle tear |

Fig. 85
Three types of vertical tears seen in the meniscus.

Clinical features
The key features of meniscal damage are:

- pain
- instability
- swelling
- locking.

Listen. Patients complain of pain in the knee and instability, especially on stairs. There is often a history of an injury while playing sports.

Look. A swelling may be seen in the infrapatellar recesses or if large in the suprapatellar pouch. The effusion must be very large before the patella rises away from the femoral condyles and a patellar tap can be elicited by balloting it back down. A swelling occurring within hours of an injury is usually due to bleeding and is a haemarthrosis. A swelling which occurs slowly is usually due to synovial fluid from the inflamed or irritated synovial lining.

Feel. There is well localised jointline tenderness usually on the medial side

Move. A block to full extension is called 'locking' and is due to trapping of an intra-articular structure, usually the displaced meniscus, within the joint. Twisting and compression manoeuvres may reproduce the pain or 'lock' or 'unlock' the joint (McMurray's test).

Diagnosis
MRI scan will show a torn meniscus but careful clinical examination will make the diagnosis in the majority of cases. Examination under anaesthesia followed by arthroscopy will make it possible to proceed to a therapeutic procedure on the same occasion. Other knee conditions with some of the same clinical features can also be seen arthroscopically. These include loose bodies (see p. 104), discoid meniscus and cystic meniscus.

Management
A large haemarthrosis should be drained urgently to relieve pain. When the diagnosis has been confirmed by arthroscopy a small meniscal tear can be trimmed or a bucket handle tear removed (Fig. 86). A peripheral detachment of the meniscus can be sewn back if several operating portals into the knee are used to place the arthroscope and other necessary instruments accurately. This minimally invasive procedure ensures that

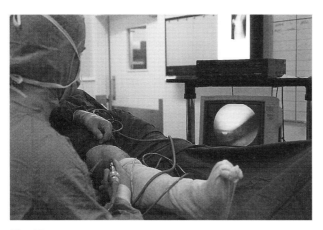

Fig. 86
Arthroscopic examination of the knee.

rehabilitation can occur in the quickest possible time. An open procedure for total meniscectomy is therefore rarely indicated today.

Complications. The articular surface of the knee may be damaged by repeated trauma from long-standing fragments of displaced meniscus.

Cruciate ligaments

The anterior cruciate ligament (ACL) arises at the anterior tibial spine, passes backwards across the knee joint to be inserted on the medial side of the lateral femoral condyle. It prevents the tibia sliding off the front of the femur.

Clinical features
A tear of the ACL is a common sporting injury (Fig. 87). Rupture of the ACL accounts for 75% of haemarthrosis associated with sports.

Listen. There is a history of a twisting injury, a direct blow behind the upper tibia or a hyper-flexion injury.

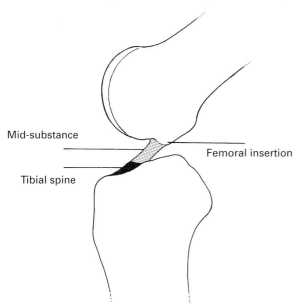

Mid-substance

Femoral insertion

Tibial spine

Fig. 87
Sites of disruption of the anterior cruciate ligament.

The patient often describes a snapping sound and sensation from the knee.

Look/feel. A haemarthrosis develops quickly.

Move. If the knee is examined before swelling and muscle spasm occur then a positive anterior drawer sign will be easily enlisted. Lachmann's test can be done if the knee joint is too swollen and painful to allow full flexion for the anterior drawer test. It involves gliding the extended tibia forwards at the knee while holding the thigh steady with the other hand. The pivot shift test, which involves moving the knee into different positions of flexion while loading the lateral compartment, can also be done but is most usefully carried out under anaesthesia.

Diagnosis
A lateral radiograph may show an avulsion of the anterior tibial spine but usually the tear is in the mid-substance of the ligament and requires MRI to visualise it. Arthroscopy of the knee will show the extent of the damage and allow drainage of the haemarthrosis.

Management
Initial treatment involves aspiration of the knee and confirmation of the diagnosis by arthroscopy.

Conservative management. Physiotherapy for the hamstrings will increase strength and the ability to stabilise the ACL deficient knee. The majority of patients will adjust their life-style to having a knee which is not stable when making sudden changes of direction at speed. Sports, such as squash, that involve cutting and turning movements are not possible but other types of physical exercise can comfortably be carried out.

Acute repair of a mid-substance tear is not possible, so patients who require a more stable knee for sporting activities need an ACL reconstruction using a prosthetic intra-articular ligament often augmented with an extra-capsular repair using a part of the iliotibial tract. In the rare cases of an avulsion of the anterior tibial spine, open reduction and internal fixation can be carried out.

Complications

- instability, especially on uneven ground; the loss of proprioception from the knee probably accounts for some of this problem.

Posterior cruciate ligament

The posterior cruciate ligament (PCL) arises on the posterior aspect of the tibia and passes anteriorly to be inserted on the lateral side of the medial femoral condyle. This ligament holds the tibia forward under the femur and prevents it dropping backwards. Injuries to the PCL are less frequently seen than ACL injuries.

Clinical features
There is a history of hyperextension or forced posterior displacement of the tibia on the femur. There is a haemarthrosis and an obvious posterior sag to the knee.

Diagnosis

MRI or arthroscopic examination confirms the diagnosis.

Management

Conservative management involves aspiration of the joint and physiotherapy to the quadriceps muscles to stabilise the knee.

Surgical management will involve open reduction and internal fixation of any avulsed bony fragment from the PCL insertion.

Complications

- Chronic instability.

Medial collateral ligament

Damage to the medial collateral ligament is usually associated with both a medial meniscus tear and damage to the anterior cruciate ligament. Injuries are usually the result of twisting forces on the knee. Isolated, pure valgus injury is unusual.

Clinical features

Clinical presentation will include:

- bruising
- swelling
- tenderness
- laxity.

Tears may be in the mid-substance of the ligament or at its origin or insertion on the femur or tibia.

Diagnosis

Radiological examination may show an avulsed bony fragment at either end of the ligament. Stress radiographs may be helpful.

Management

Conservative. Splinting in an orthosis protects the collateral ligament but allows flexion and extension.

Surgical. Reconstruction of an associated anterior cruciate ligament rupture may help to regain stability if a complex derangement of the knee is present.

Complications

- Pellegrini–Stieda syndrome (calcification and discomfort in the medial collateral ligament)
- chronic ligamentous laxity.

Lateral collateral ligament

Isolated injuries to the lateral collateral ligament are less important than medial collateral ligament injuries but may be associated with lateral capsule damage and are usually part of a complex internal derangement of the knee.

Management

A functional brace protects the ligament while allowing flexion and extension.

Complications

- Chronic ligamentous laxity.

9.3 Arthritis

Rheumatoid arthritis and osteoarthritis are both frequently seen in the knee.

Osteoarthritis

Primary osteoarthritis may develop in the knee spontaneously and is sometimes associated with a positive family history.

Secondary osteoarthritis may follow trauma, infection or intra-articular derangement of the knee, such as a ligamentous disruption or meniscectomy.

The medial side of the joint is more frequently involved than the lateral condyle.

Clinical features

Listen. There is knee pain ranging in severity from being associated only with walking, especially on stairs, to being present at rest.

Look. Classically, there is varus alignment of the joint with synovial thickening and effusion. In late cases there is a flexion contraction.

Feel. There is a swelling in the suprapatellar pouch due to effusion. Marginal osteophytes can be felt at the tibial plateau.

Move. There is loss of full extension due to flexion contraction. A valgus strain applied to the knee will correct the varus alignment and reveal laxity of the medial collateral ligament. Moving the knee produces crepitus.

Diagnosis

Radiographs show:

- joint space narrowing
- sclerosis
- subchondral cysts
- osteophytes
- varus alignment (this can be measured on a radiograph showing the entire lower limb).

Management

Conservative management includes:

- non-steroidal anti-inflammatory drugs
- walking stick
- weight reduction
- limitation of activities.

Operative management

Lavage and debridement. This sometimes gives relief. Marginal osteophytes can be trimmed and fragments of damaged articular surface and menisci washed out of the joint. This can sometimes be carried out arthroscopically. At the same time, the exact state of the articular cartilage can be assessed.

Upper tibial osteotomy. A laterally based wedge of bone at the upper tibia is removed (Fig. 88). This realigns the tibia on the femur and redistributes load across the joint, diverting high pressures from the damaged medial compartment to the undamaged lateral compartment. The osteotomy is secured with a staple. This operation is suitable for early disease in young patients.

Unicompartmental joint replacement. This replaces both the femoral and tibial sides of one half of the joint, usually the medial compartment (Fig. 89). The operation is only suitable for the early stages of the disease.

Total knee replacement. A semi-constrained surface replacement by a metal convex femoral component and a metal-backed high-density polyethylene concave tibial component is used. The prosthesis can be cemented or uncemented to the bone. The stability of the joint depends on correct tensioning of the medial and lateral collateral ligaments and on the contour of the high-density polyethylene tibial component (Fig. 90 A and B).

Arthrodesis. Surgical fusion of the joint may be appropriate for a young patient with arthritis but may also be used to salvage a knee after infection.

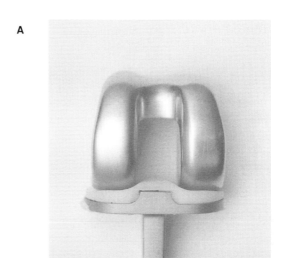

A

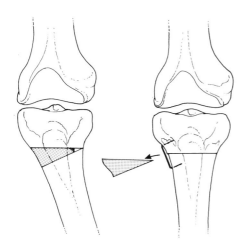

Fig. 88
Procedure of a tibial osteotomy.

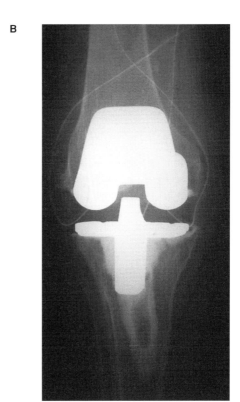

B

Fig. 90
A. Total knee prosthesis. **B.** Total knee prosthesis in situ.

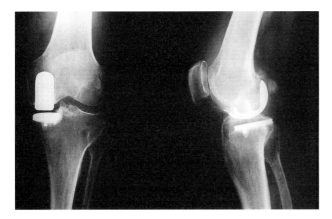

Fig. 89
Unicompartment arthroplasty.

Complications of total knee replacement

- wound dehiscence
- infection
- loosening of the components
- bone resorption
- instability
- revision surgery.

Rheumatoid arthritis (see other sections on rheumatoid)

Rheumatoid arthritis begins as inflammation of the synovium as part of an autoimmune response. The inflammation ultimately spreads to the articular cartilage and destroys it. The presence of persisting synovial effusions stretches and damages the ligaments and capsule of the joint. The joint surface becomes destroyed and the joint itself lax. This results in subluxation, deformity and painful movement.

Clinical features

- Listen — the joint is unstable; during exacerbation of the disease it becomes hot and more painful
- Look
  — swelling
  — valgus alignment
- Feel — a joint effusion may be apparent
- Move — laxity of the lateral collateral ligament.

Diagnosis

Radiographic features of rheumatoid arthritis include:

- joint space narrowing
- irregular joint surface
- marginal erosions
- valgus alignment.

Management

Medical management includes the use of both analgesics and disease-modifying drugs. Synovectomy may prevent the progression of the disease. This can be done by injection of intra-articular radioactive yttrium or as an arthroscopic procedure.

Operative. All rheumatoid patients listed for surgery must have radiographs taken of the cervical spine in flexion and extension to assess the extent of subluxation of the odontoid process as there is a risk of cord compression with cervical spike manipulation during anaesthesia.

Arthroscopic synovectomy or total joint replacement may be indicated.

Complications

- as listed for knee surgery in osteoarthritis but in rheumatoid arthritis the bone is softer and the skin thinner and more easily damaged
- Systemic manifestations: ligamentous laxity of the cervical spine may cause spinal cord compression by the odontoid process during intubation.

9.4 Loose bodies

The following may cause loose bodies to be present in the knee:

- osteochondral fractures
- osteochondritis dissecans

- separation of articular cartilage
- synovial chondromatosis
- fragments of meniscus.

Clinical features

Osteochondral fractures occur in young adults, but separation of large portions of the articular cartilage are seen in older patients. Osteochondritis dissecans is more common in boys and usually occurs between the ages of 8 and 12. The lesion is initially on the medial femoral condyle.

The patient usually complains of:
- intermittent pain
- locking and unlocking of the knee which occurs in different degrees of knee flexion
- effusion.

Diagnosis

A plain radiograph will not always show a loose body in the joint as not all are radio-opaque. The fabella (a sesamoid bone in the head of gastrocnemius) can easily be mistaken for a loose body in the joint by the unwary. A lucent line around a small part of the medial femoral condyle may be seen in osteochondritis dissecans and if a portion has become loose then a crater will be seen at the same site.

MRI and arthroscopy will visualise a lesion more clearly.

Management

A loose body in the joint can be removed arthroscopically. Such fragments often make their way to the suprapatellar pouch. An unseparated fragment can be drilled to help it heal or be pinned back in place if loose. Once the fragment has separated, it should be removed from the joint arthroscopically.

9.5 Infection

Infection may spread to the joint from osteitis in the adjacent bone. In children, the metaphysis of the proximal tibia is intra-articular. Bacteria from infection at a remote site may also be a cause. Direct intra-articular trauma is a rare cause of joint infection. Patients with diabetes mellitus are more at risk of joint infections, however. *Staphylococcus aureus* and gonococci are the common pathogens involved. A more recent cause of knee infection is arthroscopic surgery.

Clinical features

Clinical features include:
- pain
- swelling
- heat
- tenderness
- resistance to active or passive movement.

Diagnosis

There is a raised temperature, white cell count and plasma viscosity. Radiographs will show hyperaemia of the bone in the early stages.

Management

Left untreated, septic arthritis in the joint will ultimately discharge spontaneously through the skin and the joint will spontaneously fuse.

When first suspected, the joint must be aspirated and specimens sent for bacteriological examination. Antibiotics must be commenced early. If pus is aspirated from the joint then thorough irrigation via the arthroscope should be carried out. Sometimes continuous irrigation and drainage for several hours is required. In later stages of infection, arthroscopic division of adhesions is indicated.

Complications

- chronic osteitis
- spontaneous arthrodesis or fibrous ankylosis.

9.6 Intra-articular fractures

Osteochondral fractures

In young adults, shearing forces or direct trauma will produce an osteochondral fracture that may separate entirely from its bed. Such a fragment may grow in the joint because it can receive nutrition from the synovial fluid.

Management

A small fragment should be removed arthroscopically, but a large fragment should be reattached.

Tibial plateau fractures

Valgus forces directed to the knee will tear the medial collateral ligament and damage the lateral tibial plateau.

Clinical features

- Listen
  — history of an angulatory or twisting force to the knee
  — pain on the medial side of the joint
- Look
  — medial bruising
  — swelling
- — haemarthrosis may be present
- Move — valgus laxity on stressing the joint.

Diagnosis

Radiological examination may show:

- vertical split
- depression fracture (dye punch)
- comminution of the whole lateral tibial plateau

- combination of split and depression fractures.

The different types of tibial plateau fracture are shown in Figure 91.

Management

Cleavage fractures require screw fixation to restore the stability of the articular surface.

Depression fractures require elevation of the defect with a bone graft. A portion of the lateral meniscus may be found driven into the crater by the injury.

More complex fractures require elevation of the plateau and its stabilisation by a buttress plate on the

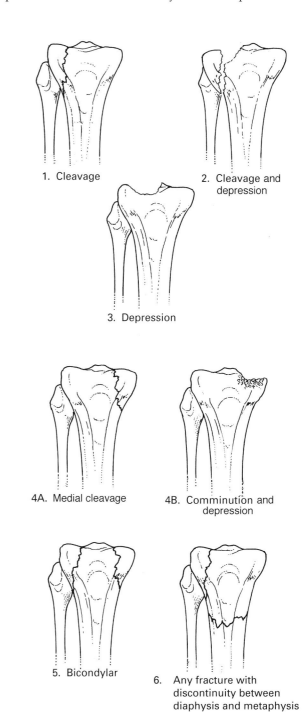

1. Cleavage

2. Cleavage and depression

3. Depression

4A. Medial cleavage

4B. Comminution and depression

5. Bicondylar

6. Any fracture with discontinuity between diaphysis and metaphysis

Fig. 91
Classification of types of tibial plateau fracture.

tibia. Bone graft is always necessary. Postoperatively, the knee is nursed in a functional brace, which allows the joint to mobilise but weight-bearing has to be avoided for 6 to 8 weeks.

Complications

- osteoarthritis requiring later total conversion to a total knee replacement
- valgus laxity
- stiff joint.

Condylar fractures of the femur

Axial angulatory forces directed across the knee may fracture the distal femur.

Clinical features

Clinical features include:

- haemarthrosis
- joint laxity.

Diagnosis

Radiological examination shows a split fracture of a single condyle or a 'Y' shaped fracture of both condyles. There may be a comminuted fracture involving both condyles.

Management

The haemarthrosis is aspirated. Plaster immobilisation may be sufficient for an undisplaced unicondylar split fracture, but accurate anatomical reduction with screw fixation to prevent subsequent displacement is preferable for more complex fractures. Postoperatively, the knee is nursed in a functional brace.

Complications

- valgus/varus angulation
- osteoarthritis.

9.7 Extensor mechanism injury

Resisted extension of the knee damages different levels of the extensor mechanism at different ages (Fig. 92).

Adolescents

Avulsion of the tibial tuberosity

A traction injury to the tibial apophysis may elevate a portion causing localised pain, tenderness and a lump. Sometimes a similar condition (Osgood–Schlatter's disease) occurs in adolescence as a result of activity but with no specific injury. In both cases, the lesion is treated by rest and a back splint.

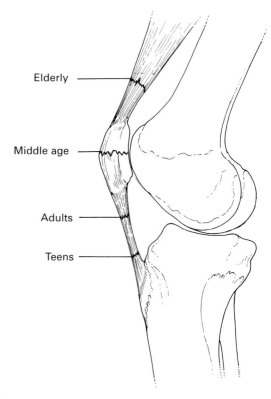

Fig. 92
Sites of rupture of the extensor mechanism at different ages.

Young patients

Ruptured patellar tendon

Straight leg raising is inhibited and a palpable gap is present. Repair of the tendon is required.

Middle life

Transverse (avulsion) fractures of the patella

A palpable gap is present in the patella, sometimes accompanied by extensive lateral and medial bruising and swelling. This indicates a probable tear in the quadriceps expansion and, if present, straight leg raising will be impossible. Repair of the fracture with tension band wire and suture of the quadriceps tear are necessary. The articular surface must be carefully restored. Quadriceps-strengthening exercises and knee flexion can begin when comfortable.

Stellate fractures of the patella

These occur from a direct blow on the patella, but the quadriceps expansion is not usually torn. There is a haemarthrosis.

A radiograph shows the extent of comminution of the fracture.

Initially the joint is aspirated. A cylinder splint may be sufficient treatment but with displaced fragments cerclage wire is required.

Elderly patients

Rupture of quadriceps tendon or rectus femoris muscle

In degenerative tissues, the muscle avulses from the tendon.

Suture is sometimes possible but the tissues are friable. Physiotherapy alone is usually sufficient to restore quadriceps function.

Complications of extensor mechanism injuries

Complications include:

- weak quadriceps and loss of straight leg raising
- a painful ossicle in the patellar tendon may be the sequela of a tibial tuberosity avulsion.

Self-assessment: questions

Multiple choice questions

1. Knee pain:
   a. Related to the medial joint line in a 60-year-old patient is, in the majority of patients, caused by a cleavage lesion of the medial meniscus
   b. At the patellar femoral joint is often a finding in adolescent females
   c. Associated with painful intermittent locking suggests the presence of an intra-articular loose body
   d. In relation to the tibial tuberosity is most commonly found in active osteoporotic females
   e. Associated with intermittent effusions suggests an acute infective synovitis

2. In acute septic arthritis:
   a. *Staphylococcus aureus* is the usual infecting organism
   b. Movement of the infected joint is restricted by adhesions
   c. Antibiotics are withheld until the appropriate sensitivities are confirmed
   d. Treatment includes joint irrigation
   e. Small joints are more commonly affected than large joints

3. Loss of both passive and active full extension in the knee is seen in:
   a. Displaced bucket handle tear of the medial meniscus
   b. Quadriceps weakness
   c. Osteoarthritis
   d. Rupture of the patellar tendon
   e. Isolated comminuted fracture of the patella

Case history

A 50-year-old window cleaner presents with pain in the medial side of his right knee. In his 20s he had a meniscectomy following a football injury.

1. What is the likely diagnosis?
2. Describe the investigations you would employ to discover more about the underlying pathology
3. Discuss the appropriate medical and surgical management of this patient

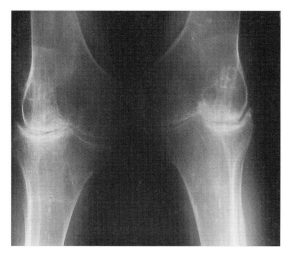

Fig. 93

Picture question

Study this radiograph of the knee (Fig. 93).

1. Indicate the abnormal radiographic features seen
2. What is the underlying diagnosis?

Short notes

1. Describe the management of a suspected case of acute septic arthritis in an adolescent's knee.
2. Discuss the pathology in the knee which may present with loss of straight leg raising.

Viva questions

1. How is a patient with a depressed fracture of the lateral tibial condyle managed?
2. Demonstrate how the knee is examined for a tear of the anterior cruciate ligament.

Self-assessment: answers

Multiple choice answers

1. a. **True.** Medial joint line pain suggests medial meniscus pathology and, in a patient of this age, a cleavage lesion caused by degeneration within the meniscus is common. The tear is horizontal in contrast to the vertical orientation of acute tears.
   b. **True.** Chondromalacia patellae is one cause of anterior knee pain commonly found in teenage girls.
   c. **True.** Locking is a mechanical block to full extension and is classically caused by a displaced meniscal tear or an intra-articular loose body, as found in osteochondritis dissecans.
   d. **False.** Pain in relation to the tibial tuberosity is associated with Osgood–Schlatter's disease, which is found in adolescent boys especially.
   e. **False.** Acute infective synovitis presents dramatically with a painful swelling with pus within the joint. Intermittent effusions are more likely to be associated with an inflammatory cause such as rheumatoid arthritis or Reiter's syndrome.

2. a. **True.**
   b. **False.** Movement is restricted by acute pain.
   c. **False.** 'Best-guess' antibiotics should be prescribed as soon as specimens have been taken for bacteriological examination.
   d. **True.** Thorough irrigation of the joint often using the arthroscope will reduce the infection.
   e. **False.** The knee and hip are the most common sites of acute septic arthritis.

3. a. **True.** A displaced bucket handle tear of the medial meniscus produces a mechanical block to passive and active extension.
   b. **False.** Full passive extension will be possible even if the quadriceps are too weak to achieve full active extension.
   c. **True.** A fixed flexion deformity of the knee from osteoarthritis will make both active and passive extension impossible.
   d. **False.** Full passive extension is still possible but active extension is not possible because of loss of continuity of the extensor mechanism.
   e. **False.** The patella fracture is painful and there is loss of continuity of the active extensor mechanism. Full passive extension, however, is possible.

Case history answer

1. The history of this patient's pain suggests secondary osteoarthritis of the medial compartment of his knee following a previous medial meniscectomy.

2. Appropriate investigations would include a standing antero-posterior and lateral radiograph to determine the extent of the disease. Arthroscopic examination would show whether early degeneration of the articular cartilage was present in the lateral compartment.

3. If the degeneration was limited to the medial compartment alone, then an upper tibial osteotomy could be used to redirect forces across the joint and off-load the medial compartment. This operation would not interfere with the stability of his knee and it would probably be safe for him to return to his employment as a window cleaner.

Picture answer

1. The radiograph of the knee shows marginal erosions, general osteoporosis, joint space narrowing and irregular joint surface. There is vagus deformity of the knees.
2. The likely diagnosis is rheumatoid arthritis.

Short notes answers

1. When septic arthritis of the joint is suspected by the clinical examination, the diagnosis can be confirmed by a raised plasma viscosity and a polymorphonuclear leucocytosis. The joint should be aspirated. The presence of opaque synovial fluid or pus confirms the diagnosis and specimens should be sent for bacteriological examination. While results are awaited, 'best-guess' antibiotics should be commenced, such as flucloxacillin and fucidin.
2. Inability to lift the leg with the knee straight implies damage to the extensor mechanism. In an adolescent, this may be caused by pain following avulsion of the tibial tuberosity. In a young patient, there may be a history of injury causing rupture of the patellar tendon or fracture to the patella. In an elderly patient, minimal trauma may cause a rupture of the quadriceps tendon or the rectus femoris muscle.

Viva answers

1. The extent of displacement of a depressed fracture of the lateral tibial plateau must be assessed by tomography or CT scan. Significantly depressed fragments require elevation and bone grafting. Buttress plate fixation may be required for large fragments.
2. The integrity of the anterior cruciate ligament is tested by pulling the tibia forward on the flexed knee. Disruption of the ligament allows the tibia to slide forward during this manoeuvre.

Foot and ankle disorders

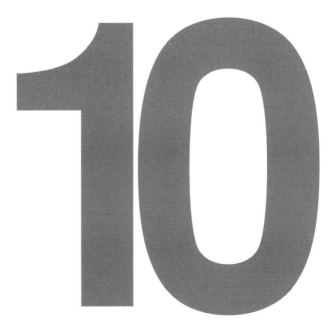

10.1 Clinical examination

Examination of the foot and ankle must include an examination of the patient walking and standing. It is important to remember to examine the patient's shoes for signs of wear on the sole and of damage to the uppers.

The patient's gait is examined while walking. With the patient standing with the feet together the posture of the foot is observed. Looking from behind, the alignment of the calcaneum can be observed and any degree of calcaneovalgus noted. The posture of the longitudinal arches can be observed. If absent, the arch will usually reconstitute when the patient stands on tiptoe. With the patient seated and the foot cradled on the examiner's knee the peripheral pulses, capillary circulation and peripheral sensation can be examined. Movements of the foot and ankle should be examined in turn. Movement occurs in the following joints:

- ankle
- subtalar
- midtarsal
- metatarsophalangeal
- interphalangeal.

At the ankle joint, only flexion and extension is possible. Subtalar movement is assessed by cupping the heel in the palm of the hand and inverting and everting the foot.

With the calcaneum fixed to the talus, inversion and eversion at the midtarsal joint can be elicited. Flexion and extension are possible at the metatarsophalangeal and interphalangeal joints.

10.2 Foot disorders

Bunions and hallux valgus

This is the most commonly occurring deformity in the foot, but it is not always symptomatic. Two distinct groups of patients usually present.

The adolescent girl. There is a strong family history of hallux valgus. The underlying abnormality is varus deformity of the first metatarsal.

The adult female. There is forefoot splaying because of ligamentous laxity. Constricting footwear may provide an additional deforming force. There may be degenerative changes in the first metatarsophalangeal joint and abnormalities of the adjacent toes. Hallux valgus is often seen in association with rheumatoid arthritis in this age group.

Clinical features
- Listen — Patients complain of rubbing or pressure over the first metatarsophalangeal joint and that their shoes feel tight.

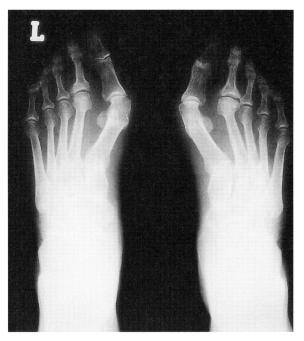

Fig. 94
Radiograph of the feet showing bilateral hallux valgus deformity. On the right there has been a previous excision of the exostosis but the underlying metatarsus primus varus remains.

- Look — There is a prominent exostosis at the first metatarsal head covered with a protective bursa. This may become inflamed or even infected. The big toe is displaced laterally, pronated and crowds the second toe so that one may override the other.
- Feel — If inflamed the bunion may be painful to touch.
- Move — Once established the valgus deformity cannot be corrected.

Diagnosis
Weight-bearing radiographs will show the extent of the deformity, the degree of subluxation of the joint and any secondary arthritic degeneration (Fig. 94).

Management
Initially, all patients should consider accepting the deformity and adapting their footwear to accommodate it. If this is not acceptable to the patient surgery can be discussed.

Adolescents. Management is usually with surgery. An osteotomy of the first metatarsal, which realigns the first ray and narrows the forefoot (Fig. 95) will correct the valgus deformity of the big toe and allow the patient to continue wearing fashionable shoes.

Adults

Orthoses. Comfortable, wide shoes that accommodate the splayed forefoot are the easiest solution. The shoe uppers are soft over the bunion and have moulded insoles to support the metatarsal heads.

Surgery

- realignment of the hallux can be achieved in patients with mild disease by a capsulorrhaphy of

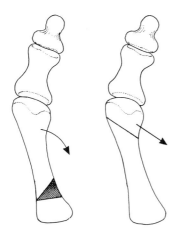

Fig. 95
Two types of osteotomy of the first metatarsal which will correct the underlying varus deformity and allow the big toe to become straighter.

the first metatarsophalangeal joint and release of the adductor hallux; an excision of the exostosis at the first metatarsal head can be included
- arthrodesis of the first metatarsophalangeal joint is indicated in more severe disease
- excision arthroplasty is suitable for older people who are less active; the base of the proximal phalanx and the exostosis are removed (Keller's operation; Fig. 96); the alignment is corrected but the big toe is now floppy and fails to provide a strong 'push off' when walking.

Complications

- local pressure effects
- bursitis.

Complications of surgery

- infection
- poor wound healing
- hallux varus or hallux erectus deformity from overcorrection
- recurrence
- altered sensation.

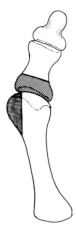

Fig. 96
Keller's arthroplasty of the first metatarsophalangeal joint.

Hallux rigidus

Some forgotten minor trauma may be the precipitating cause of this condition which affects men more than women. There is osteoarthritis of the first metatarsophalangeal joint, which causes pain and stiffness of the big toe (hallux rigidus). The changes are isolated and not part of widespread osteoarthritis.

Clinical features

- Listen
   — pain on walking, especially up hills
   — patients notice reduced stride length
   — women complain of pain when wearing high-heeled shoes
- Look — dorsal osteophyte
- Feel — local tenderness
- Move
   — first metatarsophalangeal joint is stiff
   — dorsiflexion is painful, resisted and limited.

Diagnosis

The familiar radiological features of osteoarthritis are present: sclerosis, joint space narrowing, osteophyte formation (Fig. 97).

Management

Conservative. A metatarsal bar on the shoe sole allows the patient to roll over the metatarsophalangeal joint. Low heels are comfortable.

Operative. Arthrodesis of the joint in slight dorsiflexion and adduction provide pain relief but may not

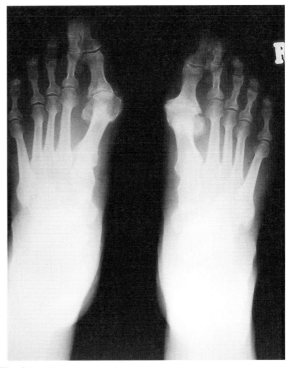

Fig. 97
Hallux valgus on the left foot and hallux rigidus on the right with radiological features of joint space narrowing, sclerosis and osteophyte formation.

accommodate varying heel sizes. Interposition arthroplasty has been used, but silicone joints tend to break down with time and cause an inflammatory synovitis.

Complications of surgery

- choice of footwear is restricted
- silicone synovitis.

Fasciitis

Fasciitis is pain at the origin of the plantar fascia where it arises from the calcaneum.

Clinical features

The main clinical features are pain on walking and localised tenderness at the calcaneum.

Diagnosis

X-ray examination sometimes shows a spur on the calcaneum.

Management

Management includes:

- heel pad
- steroid injection
- excision may be helpful, but the outcome is unpredictable.

Complications of surgery

- persisting pain
- wound infection.

Rheumatoid feet

The foot, like the hand and wrist, is often involved in rheumatoid arthritis. Ligamentous laxity following synovitis allows dorsal dislocation of the proximal phalanges on the metatarsal heads. This causes the weight-bearing pad of thick plantar skin to be drawn distally; weight-bearing, therefore, takes place through the unprotected metatarsal heads, which cause pain in the sole of the foot (Fig. 98).

Clinical features

- Listen — Patients classically complain that they are 'walking on pebbles'.
- Look — There is dorsal pressure over the prominent proximal interphalangeal joints of the toes. The metatarsal heads can be seen prominently in the sole.
- Feel — The metatarsal heads can be easily felt.
- Move — Eventually the toes cannot be corrected to their normal straight alignment.

Diagnosis

Radiological examination shows the extent of joint subluxation and of bone destruction (Fig. 99).

Management

Conservative. Wide, deep shoes with soft uppers and moulded insoles accommodate the foot comfortably.

Operative. In more severely affected patients, a forefoot arthroplasty is required. The metatarsal heads are excised, the toes realigned and the weight-bearing pad of skin, which has been drawn distally, is replaced under the metatarsal heads.

Complications. Persisting painful pressure areas in the sole are usually the result of failure to remove sufficient length from the distal metatarsals. Wound healing is occasionally prolonged.

Peripheral vascular disease

Usually the cause of peripheral vascular disease (PVD) is proximal large-vessel atheroma, but sometimes distal small-vessel disease due to diabetes is the cause. The condition in these patients is often complicated by persisting infection and ulceration, although either type of PVD may give rise to peripheral gangrene.

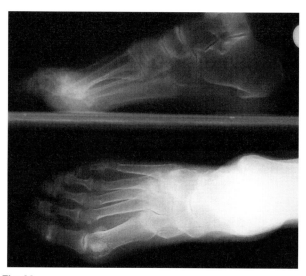

Fig. 99
This true lateral view of the foot shows the extent of the dislocation of the metatarsophalangeal joint. The metatarsal heads are touching the ground but the toes are displaced upwards and do not contribute to weight-bearing.

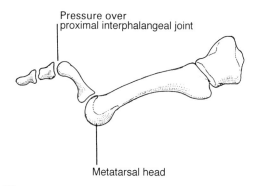

Pressure over proximal interphalangeal joint

Metatarsal head

Fig. 98
Mechanism of metatarsophalangeal joint displacement in rheumatoid arthritis.

Clinical features

- **Listen** — In large-vessel disease, the patient complains of intermittent claudication and eventually of severe constant ischaemic pain in the limb.
- **Look** — There are peripheral trophic changes, including thinning of the skin and loss of skin hair. The skin is pale and ulceration and incipient or frank gangrene may be apparent.
- **Feel** — The leg feels cold below the knee and peripheral pulses are absent (Fig. 100).
- **Move** — Elevation of the limb produces further pallor but dependency causes rubor due to verous pooling.

In diabetes, the proximal findings are not seen but peripheral infection, ulceration and dry or wet gangrene of individual toes may be present.

Diagnosis

The diagnosis can be confirmed and the level of critical ischaemia demonstrated by a non-invasive vascular assessment (NIVA). This includes:

- thermography
- pressure studies
- skin pO_2
- blood glucose.

Management

Prevention. The control of diabetes mellitus and care of the feet to avoid infection are important in diabetics. Patients with proximal atheroma are investigated by anteriogram of the affected limb and the circulation of the foot may be improved initially by a sympathectomy or in later cases by an appropriate bypass graft.

Surgery. Toes affected by dry gangrene can be allowed to demarcate and separate. In the presence of intractable pain and progressive wet gangrene, an amputation is required. Diabetic patients are well served by a Syme's amputation, which usually heals better than a midtarsal amputation. Patients with large-vessel disease usually require a below knee amputation. Well supervised prosthetic fitting and physiotherapy are required postoperatively.

Complications

- advancing gangrene
- death.

Complications following surgery

- stump breakdown occurs if the limb has been amputated too distally
- phantom limb pain.

10.3 Fractures

Ankle fractures

Injuries to the ankle are frequently seen. They are usually caused by twisting forces or angulating forces. Falls from a height often cause more severe injuries involving the distal tibial plafond. A combination of ligamentous and bony injury results.

The ligaments involved are:

- inferior tibiofibular
- anterior inferior talodeltoid
- medial collateral.

The bony margins involved are:

- medial malleolus
- lateral malleolus
- posterior surface of the tibia.

The forces that give rise to the injury can be grouped as:

- pronation and external rotation
- pronation and abduction
- supination and external rotation
- supination and adduction.

Clinical features

There is pain and swelling over one or both sides of the ankle with bruising and sometimes fracture blisters. If there is associated dislocation of the joint, there will be gross deformity, stretching of the overlying skin and loss of normal peripheral circulation and sensation.

Diagnosis

A lateral and an antero-posterior radiograph centred on the ankle mortice are required to assess the injury and to demonstrate any lateral displacement of the talus (Fig. 101).

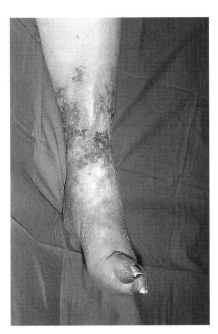

Fig. 100
Peripheral vascular disease showing rubor, trophic changes and incipient gangrene in the toes and forefoot.

Management

Conservative. Dislocation should be reduced urgently to reduce pain, relieve pressure to the peripheral circulation and nerves and to prevent ischaemia of the overlying skin. Manipulation under anaesthesia in such a way as to reverse the direction of the injuring forces will correct a displaced fracture. An above-knee plaster or patella-bearing cast is required for those injuries where rotatory control is necessary; in other patients, a well-moulded below-knee plaster is sufficient. After initial swelling has settled, partial weight-bearing can be allowed. Radiological follow-up is necessary to ensure that the fracture does not redisplace while in plaster. Immobilisation is required until the fracture heals, usually between 6 and 8 weeks.

Operative. Open reduction and internal fixation is indicated for unstable fractures. This is best done before swelling develops and must not be done through very swollen tissues as wound dehiscence will ensue. This technique restores the anatomical position of the articular surfaces and by providing rigid fixation allows early active mobilisation.

Lag screws are inserted across the fractures and the fibula is further kept out to length and stabilised by a neutralisation plate (Fig. 102). Tension band wiring is used in porotic bone in preference to screws.

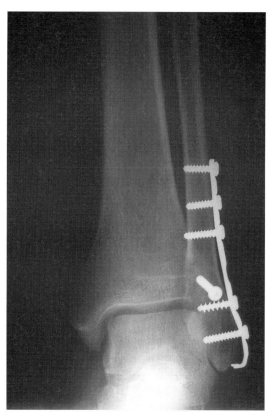

Fig. 102
The fracture has been treated with a neutralisation plate on the fibula which restores it to normal alignment and length and reduces the displacement of the talus.

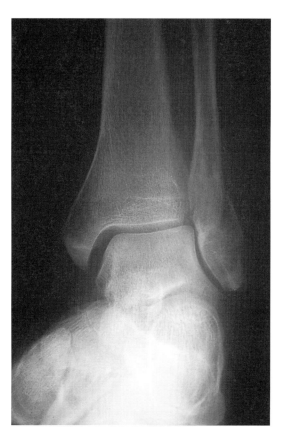

Fig. 101
Fracture of the lateral malleolus of the ankle of a young man with lateral displacement of the talus.

Complications of conservative treatment:

- malunion
- talar shift leading to
- secondary osteoarthritis.

Complications of operative treatment:

- infection
- wound dehiscence
- non-union.

Foot fractures

Talus

Forced dorsiflexion injuries to the foot can result in a fracture of the talus through either the body or the neck of the bone. Osteochondral fractures can also occur which may eventually become loose bodies in the joint.

Clinical features
Clinical presentation is with pain, swelling and bruising. If a portion of the fractured talus is displaced, it may cause pressure effects on the overlying skin.

Diagnosis
Radiological examination shows the site of the fracture but CT will give more detail.

Management

Displaced fractures require open reduction and internal fixation if avascular necrosis of the proximal fragment is to be avoided. Even with adequate treatment, there is still a substantial risk of this happening.

Complications

*   avascular necrosis of the body of the talus due to the retrograde blood supply being cut off by the fracture
*   osteoarthritis of the subtalar, talonavicular or ankle joints
*   formation of loose bodies from osteochondral fractures.

Calcaneum

A fall from a height is the usual cause of this injury and if present fractures in other sites must be sought, especially in the vertebrae, pelvis and base of the skull.

Clinical features

Clinical features include:

*   pain
*   deep bruising
*   unable to bear weight
*   fracture blisters
*   swelling.

The heel may appear wider and shorter than the opposite one.

Diagnosis

Lateral and axial radiographs (Fig. 103) are required. Three patterns of injury are described:

*   fractured 'beak' at the insertion of the Achilles tendon
*   fracture of the sustentaculum tali
*   a variety of patterns of intra-articular burst fracture through the cancellous bone.

A CT scan will show the fracture pattern more precisely.

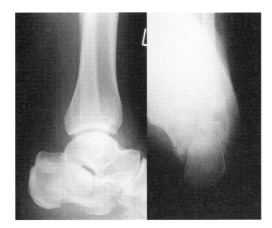

Fig. 103
Fracture of the os calcis.

Management

Elevation and exercise of the ankle and subtalar joints is appropriate management for many of these fractures. In some cases, open reduction and internal fixation with a bone graft is possible, but adequate fixation is technically difficult and wound breakdown is common. After either procedure weight-bearing is prohibited for at least 8 weeks.

Complications

*   persisting pain
*   subtalar arthritis, requiring subsequent fusion of the subtalar joint.

10.4 Ankle disorders

Achilles tendon injury

Rupture of the Achilles tendon usually occurs in patients in middle age during the course of some strenuous activity such as running or playing squash.

Clinical features

*   Listen — A sudden movement of the ankle is followed by acute severe pain such that patients frequently think they have been hit in the back of the calf.
*   Look — The gap in the tendon may be visible beneath the skin before swelling develops.
*   Feel — Palpation reveals a gap in the tendon at the ankle.
*   Move — There may be loss of normal plantar flexion when the calf is squeezed (Symons' test).

Diagnosis

The clinical features are usually convincing, but sometimes tenderness is located in the mid-calf, in which case a partial rupture of the medial head of the gastrocnemius or a rupture of the plantaris tendon must be suspected.

Management

Conservative. An equinus above-knee cast is worn for the first 4 weeks before changing to a cast in plantigrade. After a further 4 weeks, a heel raise is fitted to the patient's ordinary shoes and exercises are begun.

Operative. Operative repair achieves a quicker result but the outcome in the long term is only marginally better than with conservative treatment.

Complications

*   rerupture
*   poor spring during toe-off
*   scar sensitivity after operative repair
*   stiffness.

Self-assessment: questions

Multiple choice questions

1. Acceptable lines of management for metatarsalgia and dorsal dislocation of the metatarsophalangeal joints in rheumatoid disease include:
   a. Amputation at the tarsometatarsal joint level
   b. Excision of the metatarsal heads
   c. Excision of the proximal phalanges
   d. The prescription of soft, deep shoes
   e. Excision of the intermetatarsal neuromas

2. Below-knee amputation:
   a. Walking requires less energy following this than following an above-knee amputation
   b. Is recommended for those patients who have 50° fixed flexion of the knee
   c. Is best performed utilising a long posterior fasciocutaneous flap
   d. Plaster of Paris is an accepted type of postoperative dressing
   e. Requires 3 months of healing before a prosthetic limb is applied

3. Symptoms from hallux valgus in a middle-aged female may be treated satisfactorily by:
   a. Fusion of the first metatarsophalangeal joint
   b. Plaster splintage for 6 weeks
   c. Tendon transfer
   d. Proximal hemiphalangectomy of the proximal phalanx
   e. Amputation of the second toe

4. Infected gangrene in the foot of a diabetic patient may result from:
   a. Disease of large blood vessels
   b. Disease of small blood vessels
   c. Neuropathy
   d. Injury
   e. Deep infection

Case history

> A 60-year-old lady complains of pain in her first metatarsophalangeal joint on walking. A diagnosis of hallux rigidus is suspected.

1. What clinical features would be expected?
2. What treatment would be recommended?
3. What information regarding postoperative limitations should the patient be given before commencing surgery?

Picture question

Study the radiograph of this young man's ankle fracture (Fig. 104).

1. How would you describe the injuries?
2. In what direction has the injuring force been applied?
3. Describe how this fracture would usually be treated

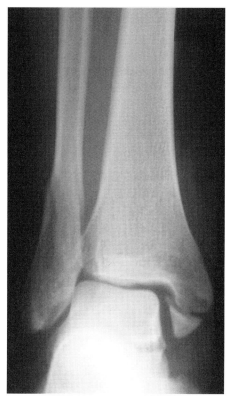

Fig. 104
Ankle injury in a young man.

Short notes

1. List the advantages and disadvantages of open reduction and internal fixation of ankle fractures.
2. Describe the natural history of a fracture of the neck of the talus. What is the method of treatment of choice?

Viva questions

1. Demonstrate how to examine a limb for peripheral vascular disease.
2. Describe the clinical findings to be seen on examination of the rheumatoid foot.

Self-assessment: answers

Multiple choice answers

1. a. **False.** While amputation at the metatarsophalangeal joint level may be required for an isolated toe in occasional circumstances, amputation at the mid-foot or tarsometatarsal joint level is not appropriate.
   b. **True.** An excision of the metatarsal heads will shorten the length of the ray and allow the displaced proximal phalanges to be returned to normal alignment.
   c. **True.** This operation removes the displaced phalanges but shortens the toe.
   d. **True.** A non-operative approach would be the provision of soft, deep shoes which accommodate the toes in the deformed position.
   e. **False.** The pain of metatarsalgia in the rheumatoid foot is caused by a dorsal dislocation of the proximal phalanges and not an intermetatarsal neuroma.

2. a. **True.**
   b. **False.** The presence of an uncorrectable fixed flexion deformity of the knee precludes a below-knee amputation and amputation at the above-knee site is necessary.
   c. **True.** The provision of a posterior fasciocutaneous flap allows the anterior suture line to be more proximal and away from the stump end.
   d. **True.** Postoperative oedema in the stump is best controlled by a light plaster of Paris dressing.
   e. **False.** Early temporary prosthetic fitting is encouraged to allow the patient to stand upright and begin mobilising as soon after surgery as possible.

3. a. **True.** This operation maintains the length of the first ray and controls the position of the hallux.
   b. **False.** The deforming forces have produced an established deformity that will not be corrected by splintage.
   c. **False.** This operation may be more appropriate in younger patients.
   d. **True.** This operation corrects the valgus deformity but shortens and weakens the big toe.
   e. **True.** In some patients, more space can be made for the deformed hallux by amputating the adjacent toe.

4. a. **True.**
   b. **True.**
   c. **True.** Neuropathy associated with diabetes means that trivial injuries in the feet are unrecognised and infection is able to develop.
   d. **True.**
   e. **True.**

Case history answer

1. In hallux rigidus, the clinical findings include the presence of a dorsal osteophyte at the metatarsal head, stiffness of the joint and pain on attempted movement.
2. Treatment of choice is an arthrodesis of the first metatarsophalangeal joint in sufficient degree of dorsiflexion to permit the patient to wear shoes with a low heel.
3. Prior to surgery the patient should understand that it will not be possible to wear shoes with high heels once the angle of the arthrodesis has been set.

Picture answer

1. The radiograph of this ankle fracture shows a spiral fracture of the lateral malleolus and a transverse avulsion fracture of the medial malleolus.
2. This is an supination–external rotation injury. The fracture is unstable and lateral migration of the talus is a likely sequelae.
3. The fracture is best treated in a young adult by open reduction and internal fixation. Lag screws are used to secure the medial malleolar fragment and a one-third tubular neutralisation plate controls the lateral malleolus and restores it to full length (Fig. 105).

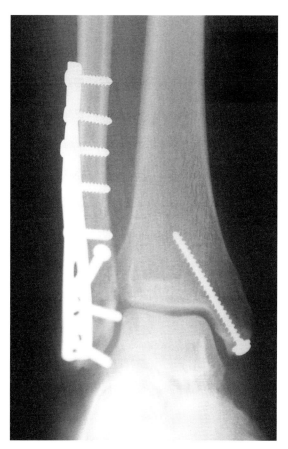

Fig. 105
The fracture has been treated by internal fixation with a lag screw to the medial malleolus and neutralisation plate to the fibula.

Short notes answers

1. The advantages of open reduction and internal fixation of an ankle fracture are:

   - anatomical reduction
   - early mobilisation
   - the avoidance of malunion, which would lead to point loading and osteoarthritic degeneration of the joint.

   The disadvantages of surgically correcting a fracture are:

   - risk of infection
   - delayed or non-union
   - implant failure
   - it may be necessary to remove the fixation devices later because of local pressure effects or persisting pain.

2. The natural history of a fracture of the neck of the talus is for the proximal fragment to undergo avascular necrosis. If this occurs, then secondary osteoarthritic degeneration of the ankle joint will follow. The treatment of choice for fractures of the neck of the talus is anatomical reduction as an open procedure and internal fixation by lag screws.

Viva answers

1. When examining a limb for peripheral vascular disease, the limb is observed for trophic changes in the skin and loss of hair-bearing capacity. There may be ulceration and inflammation or infection. Peripheral pulses are absent. The limb feels cold. Elevation of the leg produces a marked pallor and dependency produces redness.

2. The rheumatoid foot classically shows hallux valgus and dorsal dislocation of the metatarsophalangeal joints. Examination of the sole shows the metatarsal heads to be prominent and covered only by superficial skin. The thick weight-bearing pad of skin has been pulled distally. The metatarsophalangeal joints may have subluxated or be dislocated, and passive reduction may be impossible. There may be callosities or pressure effects over the dorsum of the proximal interphalangeal joint of these toes. Peripheral circulation and sensation should be examined. The presence of vasculitis in the toes should be noted.

Ear, nose and throat

Section

2

The ear

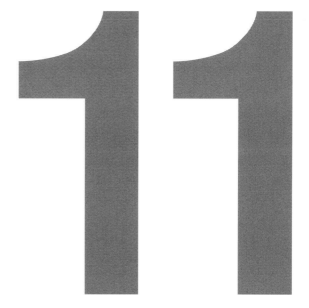

11.1 Anatomy and physiology

The ear is subdivided into three parts (Fig. 106):

- external
- middle
- inner.

External ear

The external ear is composed of the auricle, the external auditory canal and the tympanic membrane. The ear canal skin covers bone medially and cartilage laterally. Epithelial migration of the skin of the ear canal is from medial to lateral. Laterally the skin contains hair follicles and ceruminous glands. The tympanic membrane has an upper thin part, the pars flaccida, and a lower thicker part, the pars tensa (Fig. 107). The malleus handle is embedded in the substance of the tympanic membrane and the long process of the incus may be seen deep to the tympanic membrane postero-superiorly.

Middle ear

The middle ear is connected to the nasopharynx via the Eustachian tube and also posteriorly to the mastoid air cells. The ossicular chain comprises three ossicles, the malleus, incus and stapes. They transmit vibration from the tympanic membrane to the inner ear. The stapedius and tensor tympani muscles are attached to the stapes and malleus, respectively. The facial nerve lies in a narrow bony tunnel (Fallopian canal) in the temporal bone and may be damaged by disease of the surrounding bone.

Inner ear

The inner ear comprises the cochlea, concerned with hearing, and the semicircular canals, utricle and saccule, concerned with balance. These structures relay neural impulses to the central auditory and central vestibular systems, respectively. The central vestibular system also receives and coordinates proprioceptive and visual information.

Common presenting complaints are:

- hearing loss
- tinnitus
- vertigo
- aural discharge
- otalgia.

11.2 Clinical examination

Ear examination involves inspection of the surrounding skin as well as of the ear canal and tympanic membrane with a battery powered auroscope.

Initially the ear is inspected for scars, both postaural and endaural.

To straighten the ear canal for otoscopic examination in adults, gently pull the auricle up and back. In children, gently pull the auricle straight back and if necessary slightly downwards. The otoscope should be held like a pen. This initially feels awkward but allows easier more gentle inspection. Remember that in some patients not all of the tympanic membrane can be seen. In particular the antero-inferior part of the tympanic membrane may be obscured by a prominent anterior canal wall. The pneumatic attachment to the auroscope can be used to assess the mobility of the tympanic membrane (Seigeloscopy).

A 512 Hz tuning fork is used for Rinne and Weber hearing tests.

Investigations

Tests of hearing

Assessment of hearing is made initially by noting the patient's response to a normal conversational voice.

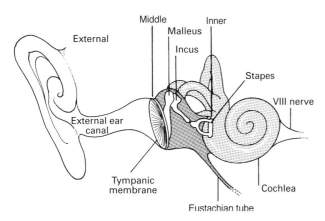

Fig. 106
Anatomy of the ear.

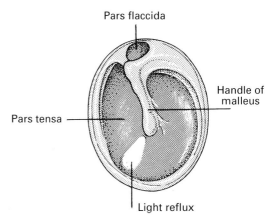

Fig. 107
The tympanic membrane.

Hearing loss caused by disease of the external or middle ear is termed conductive hearing loss, that caused by disease of the inner ear is termed sensory hearing loss and that caused by the disease of the auditory nerve is termed neural hearing loss. In practice, it is often difficult to distinguish the last two types of hearing loss and they are commonly referred to as sensorineural or perceptive hearing loss.

Tuning fork tests

The 512 Hz tuning fork is struck on the tester's knee or elbow and air and bone conduction hearing is tested.

The Rinne test compares air conduction with bone conduction in the test ear. The tuning fork is placed lateral to the ear to test air conduction and on the mastoid process to test bone conduction. In the normal ear, air conduction should be greater than bone conduction. This is called a positive Rinne test. It may also indicate sensorineural hearing loss. If bone conduction is greater than air conduction, a negative Rinne test, conductive hearing loss is present in the test ear.

A false negative Rinne occurs in the test ear when this ear has a severe sensorineural hearing loss. This is because bone conduction is heard in the opposite ear when the tuning fork is applied to the mastoid of the ear with the sensorineural loss. The introduction of a blocking sound to the non-test ear (masking) is required.

The Weber test compares bone conduction in both ears. The tuning fork is placed in the midline of the skull. If the sound is heard in midline the test is normal. In an abnormal test, the sound lateralises to the side of conductive hearing loss and away from the side of sensorineural loss.

Audiometric tests

These may be subjective or objective.

Subjective. Pure tone audiometry measures hearing over a range of frequencies in each ear by air and bone conduction. Speech audiometry tests speech reception thresholds and speech discrimination.

Objective. Impedance audiometry detects middle ear disease such as otitis media with effusion and can also assess the condition of the ossicular chain. Evoked response audiometry measures evoked potentials from brain stem, mid-brain and auditory cortex. These may be used to determine auditory thresholds, and brain stem audiometry is a useful screening test for retro-cochlear disease such as acoustic neuroma.

Tests of balance

Maintenance of balance involves integration of information provided by the inner ears, the eyes and the proprioceptive organs. This integration occurs in the central vestibular system. Disruption of the integrity of the vestibular system results in vertigo, which is a hallucination of movement of self or of surroundings.

The labyrinths send nerve impulses to the brain stem and their function is analogous to that of a twin-engined aeroplane. Loss of function of one end organ can be compensated by central mechanisms, but acute loss is characterised by vertigo and nystagmus. Compensation occurs rapidly in the young, but in the elderly complete compensation may not be achieved.

The integrity of the vestibular apparatus may be tested in various ways. In the Hallpike test, the patient sits on an examination couch in the erect position. The patient's head is then brought briskly to hang over the end of the couch and the eyes are examined for nystagmus. The patient returns to the original position and the test is repeated with the head rotated to the left and again with the head rotated to the right. The fistula test is performed by applying positive pressure to the column of air in the ear canal, either by digital pressure on the tragus or using a pneumatic otoscope. If a fistula to the inner ear is present, the patient will complain of imbalance or vertigo and nystagmus may be observed.

Caloric stimulation of the inner ear by irrigation of the ear canal by warm (44°C) or cold (30°C) air or water results in nystagmus which may be measured to assess the integrity of the labyrinth being stimulated.

Imaging

The middle and inner ears as well as the posterior cranial fossa may be imaged by conventional CT scanning and MRI scanning.

Aids to hearing

A hearing aid has three components: a microphone, an amplifier and an earphone. Sound is conducted to the ear via an ear-mould or very occasionally through the skull via a bone vibrator. 'In the ear' aids and 'in canal' aids are available commercially and 'in the ear' aids are now being introduced in the UK through the NHS. Larger body-worn aids are sometimes helpful for those who have difficulty manipulating the small controls of conventional hearing aids. All hearing aids have an O/T/M switch. O is for off; M is for microphone and T is for switching the microphone to the telecoil for use with an induction loop system. Frequency adjustment may also be made with the H (high) and L (low) tone screw.

Even the most sophisticated hearing aid is essentially an amplifier. Patients with conductive hearing loss do well with properly adjusted hearing aids, but patients with poor speech discrimination tend to do less well. Patients fitted with hearing aids should be reviewed routinely to identify problems as they arise. Other devices such as telephone amplifiers, loud doorbells and flashing alarm lights can improve the quality of life of the hard of hearing. Cochlear implants are appropriate only for patients who are profoundly deaf in both ears. Cochlear implantation is now being undertaken in both adults and children.

11.3 Diseases of the ear

The external ear

Infection

Infection is also known as external otitis, often called swimmer's ear, and is caused by opportunistic bacteria or fungi. This condition is treated by local debridement and ear drops, which usually contain a steroid in combination with an antibacterial or antifungal agent.

Obstruction

Osteomas (solitary benign bony tumours) and exostoses (diffuse, usually multiple, bony swellings) narrow the ear canal. They may not produce symptoms, but if they result in wax impaction and external otitis they need to be surgically removed.

Foreign bodies in the ear canal usually occur in toddlers. If not easily removed, referral to an otologist is required and occasionally general anaesthesia is needed. More damage may be done to the ear by unskilled attempts at removal than by the presence of the foreign body itself.

Wax impaction can obstruct the ear. The wax may be softened by use of bicarbonate, olive oil or almond oil ear drops. Once soft, wax may be removed by syringing, but if perforation (current or healed) is suspected, a wax curette should be used. Occasionally wax removal under magnification using the operating microscope is necessary.

The middle ear

Infection

Acute otitis media is most common in young children and it is usually caused by *Haemophilus influenzae* infection. It presents with otalgia, hearing loss and, if the tympanic membrane ruptures, discharge. It is usually preceded by an upper respiratory tract infection and antibiotics are usually given. Tympanic membrane perforations following this condition usually heal spontaneously. Should the perforation fail to heal spontaneously, surgical repair of the tympanic membrane (myringoplasty) may be undertaken. If the ossicular chain has been damaged, it may be repaired by ossiculoplasty. Myringoplasty has a very high success rate — usually over 90%. Temporalis fascia is the most commonly used graft material. Ossiculoplasty results are much less predictable as the grafts or prostheses used to reconstruct the ossicular chain are subject to infection, migration and extrusion.

Otitis media with effusion is common in children. It is associated with a conductive hearing loss and may present as slow speech development, poor performance at school and disruptive behaviour. Fluid accumulates in the middle ear space as a result of Eustachian tube blockage. The fluid is usually sterile. The condition is usually self-limiting but if persistent may require myringotomy, possibly with the insertion of a grommet to maintain ventilation. Sometimes adenoidectomy is required in addition. Depending on the design, grommets tend to extrude spontaneously in six to twelve months. Occasionally grommets require to be removed surgically.

Chronic suppurative otitis media is associated with tympanic membrane perforation and aural discharge. There may be associated external otitis. Gram-negative organisms are usually involved. It may respond to medical therapy, but if cholesteatoma is present, surgery is usually required.

Cholesteatoma results from the presence of keratinising squamous epithelium in the middle ear. It presents as a chronic, smelly aural discharge. The epithelium invades the underlying bone and may result in complications such as intracranial infection, labyrinthitis and facial nerve paralysis. Mastoid surgery is required to remove disease and to prevent development of complications. Such surgery may result in the creation of a mastoid cavity which will require periodic debridement by the otologist throughout the patient's life. Nowadays it is sometimes possible to remove cholesteatoma without the creation of a mastoid cavity (intact canal wall procedure).

Hereditary disease

Otosclerosis results in fixation of the stapes footplate, with resultant conductive hearing loss. The inner ear is sometimes involved with associated sensory hearing loss. The condition is familial and is transmitted by autosomal dominant inheritance with incomplete penetrance. The incidence is likely to be similar in both sexes, but because of hormonal influences it presents twice as commonly in females. Treatment is by hearing aid or operation (stapedotomy), which replaces the immobile stapes with a prosthesis. Stapedotomy is generally a very successful operation resulting in elimination of the conductive hearing loss (closure of the air–bone gap on the audiogram). Occasionally damage to the inner ear occurs, resulting in sensorineural hearing loss, tinnitus and vertigo. These risks need to be explained to the patient. Because of them, stapedotomy is not undertaken in an only hearing ear.

Tumours

Tumours of the external, middle and inner ears are uncommon. Glomus tumours involving the middle ear or the base of the skull may present as unilateral pulsatile tinnitus. They are treated by surgery, sometimes preceded by embolisation.

Trauma

Minor trauma results from foreign bodies being

inserted into the ear canal in an attempt to remove wax. This usually results in further wax impaction.

The inner ear

Hearing loss of old age

Presbycusis is the hearing loss of old age. Higher frequencies of hearing tend to be affected first and patients have difficulty hearing female voices and background noise. There is associated deterioration of the central auditory system. A hearing aid is usually helpful but requires quiet surroundings to function best.

Noise-induced hearing loss

Noise-induced hearing loss may result from industrial or recreational noise exposure. Initially the hearing loss is often reversible, but with repeated exposure, permanent damage occurs. The loss is often greatest initially at 4 and 6 kHz. Avoidance of hazardous noise exposure is best, but if this is not possible adequate hearing protection should be worn.

Trauma

Trauma to the temporal bone may result in conductive, sensory or mixed hearing loss with or without facial paralysis. The inner ear is well protected in the petrous temporal bone and fractures of this bone usually result from considerable force, often associated with loss of consciousness.

Drugs

Ototoxic drugs, e.g. aminoglycosides, may affect the auditory, vestibular or both parts of the inner ear. Most ototoxic drugs induce permanent changes in the inner ear, but a few drugs such as aspirin and quinine result in reversible damage.

Sudden hearing loss

Sudden sensorineural hearing loss results from viral or vascular damage to the inner ear. Hearing loss may be temporary, but in some patients it is permanent and profound.

Tumour

Acoustic neuroma, more properly termed vestibular schwannoma, commonly presents with unilateral tinnitus and hearing loss. Imbalance is common but true vertigo is unusual. Any unexplained, progressive unilateral or asymmetrical sensorineural hearing loss should be investigated for possible acoustic neuroma. MRI scan is the definitive investigation, but brain stem audiometry is a useful screen. Ideally acoustic neuromas are detected when small and are treated surgically by removal with minimal morbidity. The approach to the tumour may be neurosurgical, otologic or combined. In elderly unfit patients with minimal symptoms, slowly growing tumours may best be left untreated. Serial MRI scans allow tumour growth to be assessed over time.

Menière's disease

Menière's disease is characterised by fluctuating sensory hearing loss, tinnitus and vertigo. There is often an associated feeling of fullness in the affected ear. The aetiology is unknown. The disease is usually unilateral, but with time the other ear may become affected. There is no clear evidence that the natural course of the condition is affected by medical therapy. Various operations are described for severe, intractable disease. Destructive operations, such as labyrinthectomy and division of the vestibular nerve are effective in controlling symptoms. Labyrinthectomy, by definition, destroys the hearing function of the inner ear and is only undertaken when the affected ear has very poor hearing. Non-destructive procedures include decompression and shunting of the endolymphatic sac, but the efficacy of such procedures remains in doubt.

Vertigo

Vestibular neuronitis presents as acute vertigo with no associated hearing loss or tinnitus. It is self-limiting over a period of days or weeks.

Benign positional vertigo results from semicircular canal dysfunction and is characterised by episodic vertigo consequent upon adopting a given head position. It may occur after head injury and is usually self-limiting after some months.

11.4 Miscellaneous conditions

Diseases of the facial nerve

Bell's palsy is an isolated, idiopathic lower motor neurone paralysis of the facial nerve, which is suspected to be caused by herpes viral infection. The eye becomes vulnerable if it does not close completely and tear production may be diminished. The patient should be advised about the need for eye protection. Patients with incomplete Bell's palsy recover spontaneously and require no treatment. Those with complete paralysis require investigation and possibly steroid therapy. Other disease that may result in lower motor neurone facial paralysis, such as cholesteatoma, acoustic neuroma and parotid malignancy, must be excluded.

Ramsay–Hunt syndrome results from herpes zoster involvement of the inner ear. It is characterised by hearing loss, vertigo and facial nerve palsy. Recovery of the facial nerve palsy may be incomplete. Systemic antiherpetic therapy may be helpful in relieving symptoms.

Trauma to the facial nerve may occur at any point along its course. A stab of the cheek may result in peripheral division of the nerve, while fractures of the temporal bone may damage it more proximally. Early surgical repair with grafting, if indicated, offers the best chance of recovery in a facial nerve which has been divided.

Tinnitus

Tinnitus, commonly described as buzzing or hissing noises in the ears or head, is common and usually associated with hearing loss. Resolution of the hearing loss may improve the tinnitus because of the masking effect of previously unheard sounds. Bilateral tinnitus is rarely of serious significance and patients should be reassured. Unilateral tinnitus requires further investigation. Background noise or a masker often helps to suppress the tinnitus. Anxiety and depression should be treated appropriately.

Referred otalgia

Pain felt in the ear in the absence of any ear disease is very common. Although the teeth and temporo-mandibular joints are common sources, disease of the tongue and throat must be excluded. Occasionally pain is referred from the thyroid (de Quervain's thyroiditis) or trachea.

Self-assessment: questions

Multiple choice questions

1. Recognised complications of acute otitis media include:
   a. Tympanic membrane perforation
   b. Facial nerve paralysis
   c. Temporal lobe abscess
   d. Sensorineural hearing loss
   e. Recurrent tonsillitis

2. Conductive hearing loss is a symptom of:
   a. Clinical otosclerosis
   b. Menière's disease
   c. Cholesteatoma
   d. Bell's palsy
   e. Acoustic neuroma

Case history

A 43-year-old school teacher complains of tinnitus and mild hearing loss affecting the left ear for several months. She has also noticed slight unsteadiness when getting up to go to the bathroom in the dark. Her ears are clinically normal on examination. Using the 512 Hz tuning fork, the Rinne test is positive bilaterally; the Weber is heard in the right ear.

1. What type of hearing loss does the patient most likely have?
2. What further physical examination would be appropriate?
3. What audiological tests should be done?
4. What radiological investigations should be undertaken?
5. What is the most potentially serious condition that could cause these symptoms?
6. What is the treatment of this condition?

Picture question

Figure 108 shows the ear of a 52-year-old female complaining of left-sided otalgia and facial weakness.

1. What abnormalities do you see?
2. What has produced these lesions?
3. What else may the patient complain of?
4. What is the appropriate treatment?
5. What long-term sequelae may result from this condition?

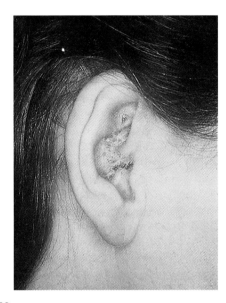

Fig. 108
The ear of a 52-year-old female complaining of left-sided otalgia and facial weakness. (Reproduced courtesy of Mr R S Dhillon FRCS.)

Short notes

Write short notes on the following:

1. referred otalgia
2. complications of cholesteatoma
3. management of Bell's palsy
4. otitis externa
5. sensorineural hearing loss

Self-assessment: answers

Multiple choice answers

1. a. **True.** Rupture of the tympanic membrane in acute otitis media is often associated with bloodstained purulent discharge and relief of pain.
   b. **True.** Facial nerve paralysis may occur when the bony covering of the nerve in its passage through the middle ear is thin or absent.
   c. **True.** Possible, but extremely rare. Intracranial complications are much more likely to occur when cholesteatoma is present.
   d. **False.** Conductive hearing loss is a feature of acute otitis media. Sensorineural hearing loss implies involvement of the labyrinth.
   e. **False.** Acute otitis media results from infection ascending from the nasopharynx. Recurrent tonsillitis may occur in association with acute otitis media but is not a complication.

2. a. **True.** Progressive conductive hearing loss is the cardinal feature of clinical otosclerosis.
   b. **False.** Menière's disease is characterised by a fluctuating, progressive sensory hearing loss.
   c. **True.** Cholesteatoma damages and frequently destroys parts of the ossicular chain. Hearing may be preserved by transmission of sound through the cholesteatoma. The conductive hearing loss may, therefore, be greater following surgery to eradicate cholesteatoma.
   d. **False.** Bell's palsy is not associated with hearing loss.
   e. **False.** Acoustic neuroma is characterised by a neural (retrocochlear) hearing loss that is unilateral. The patient often notices tinnitus before hearing loss.

Case history answers

1. The presence of unsteadiness suggests a possible peripheral vestibular disorder. The tuning fork tests suggest either a left sensorineural hearing loss or a mild right conductive loss. Given that the patient complains of left-sided hearing loss, it is most likely to be sensorineural.

2. Cranial nerves V and VII should be examined as these may be involved in cerebello-pontine angle lesions such as acoustic neuroma. Evidence of spontaneous, gaze and positional nystagmus should be sought. Cerebellar and posterior column function should be assessed. The head and neck should be auscultated for cranial and cervical bruits.

3. Pure tone and speech audiometry should be undertaken. Given the nature of the symptoms, acoustic neuroma is a possible diagnosis and, therefore, auditory brain stem responses should be assessed, comparing the latency of the response between the two sides. Vestibular function testing in the form of electronystagmography would also be appropriate. This should include caloric testing, which allows the function of each labyrinth to be assessed independently.

4. The most appropriate radiological investigation depends on available facilities. The 'gold standard' for detecting acoustic neuroma is MRI and in centres where this is readily available MRI of the posterior cranial fossa will rapidly exclude life-threatening retrocochlear disease. Plain films of the internal auditory canals and tomograms may show evidence of widening of the internal canal and demineralisation of bone. CT scanning is likely to show a large cerebello-pontine angle tumour but may miss a small mass lesion.

5. The most potentially serious condition that could cause these symptoms is a cerebello-pontine angle tumour. Most such tumours are acoustic neuromas, which in fact are tumours of Schwann cell origin from the superior vestibular nerve. Other lesions such as meningioma, arachnoid cyst and facial nerve neuroma may present in this area.

6. If an acoustic neuroma is detected in an otherwise healthy 43-year-old patient, surgical removal is the treatment of choice. Nowadays, this may be achieved without damage to the facial nerve and sometimes it is possible to preserve some hearing. In an older person with a small tumour, it may be appropriate not to treat.

Picture answer

1. There are vesicles and crusts involving the auricle.
2. These lesions are produced by the herpes zoster virus.
3. The patient may complain of hearing loss and vertigo.
4. Powerful analgesics are required. The patient may be confined to bed because of vertigo. Antiviral therapy such as acylovir may be used.
5. In contrast to Bell's palsy, where 90% of patients will recover good facial function, only about 60% do so following the Ramsay–Hunt syndrome. Post-herpetic neuralgia may be a problem and hearing may not return to normal.

Short notes answers

1. Most referred otalgia is of dental or temporo-mandibular joint origin. In the absence of other symptoms, dental referral is indicated. Referred otalgia is common following tonsillectomy via the glossopharyngeal nerve. Nevertheless the ear

should be inspected to rule out acute infection. Referred otalgia may be the sign of more serious disease such as carcinoma of the tongue base or hypopharynx and occasionally is the presenting feature of sub-acute thyroiditis (de Quervain's) disease.

2. Complications of cholesteatoma include damage to the structures in the middle ear, such as the ossicular chain and the facial nerve. The inner ear may be involved resulting in labyrinthitis. The most serious complications involve intracranial spread of infection and include meningitis and intracranial abscesses such as extradural and subdural abscesses. Abscesses may also involve the temporal lobe and cerebellum.

3. Bell's palsy is a diagnosis of exclusion and other causes of lower motor neurone facial palsy such as cholesteatoma and parotid malignancy must be excluded. If the paralysis is incomplete and does not progress, prognosis is excellent and no specific treatment beyond reassurance and eye protection is required. If the face is totally paralysed, a course of steroids for 5 to 10 days is usually given. In 90% of all patients with Bell's palsy, good facial function will be regained. Aberrant reinnervation may result in synkinesis and mass movement.

4. Otitis externa results from infection of the skin of the ear canal by opportunistic bacteria such as *Pseudomonas* and *Proteus* spp. and sometimes by fungi such as *Candida albicans* and *Aspergillus niger*. The infection tends to occur more commonly in swimmers and during warm humid weather. The mainstay of treatment is debridement of the ear canal with the removal of debris and instillation of appropriate medication, which is usually antibiotic and steroid-containing ear-drops. If the condition is chronic or recurrent, underlying causes such as more generalised skin problems or diabetes mellitus should be considered.

5. Sensorineural hearing loss may be congenital or acquired. Management is dependent on age, presentation and degree of severity. Accurate assessment of auditory thresholds by appropriate audiometric testing is mandatory and should be followed by appropriate habilitation or rehabilitation as required.

The nose and paranasal sinuses

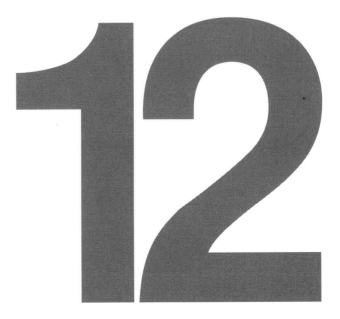

12.1 Anatomy and physiology

The nose

The external nose (Fig. 109)
The upper one-third of the external nose is bony and is covered by mobile thin skin. The lower two-thirds is cartilaginous and is covered by tightly adherent skin that contains multiple sebaceous glands.

The nasal cavities
These pass in an antero-posterior (not superior) direction in the skull for 6 to 7 cm in the adult. They are divided by a bony and cartilaginous nasal septum (Fig. 110), which is rarely absolutely in the mid-line. The major features of the lateral nasal wall (Fig. 111) are the upper, middle and inferior turbinates, which contain erectile tissue. The cavities are lined by respiratory epithelium that is thick over the turbinates and thinner over the septum. The nose has a rich blood supply from both the external and internal carotid arterial systems. Some nasal venous drainage passes intracranially to the cavernous sinuses.

Function
Besides being the olfactory organ, the nose warms and humidifies the inspired air. Particulate matter is trapped anteriorly at the nasal vestibule by the nasal vibrissae. Smaller particles adhere to the mucus blanket that lines the nasal mucosa and are transported posteriorly by mucociliary activity and swallowed. The olfactory epithelium is located high in the nasal cavity below the cribriform plates. Nasal obstruction from any cause results in reduced air flow and reduced sense of smell. Nasal obstruction may also result in loss of vocal resonance. Excess nasal patency also alters voice quality.

Paranasal sinuses

These are paired structures (Fig. 112) comprising:

- anterior group: frontal, maxillary and anterior ethmoid sinuses; these all drain to the middle meatus below the inferior turbinate
- posterior group: posterior ethmoids drain to the middle meatus; sphenoid sinuses.

Not all paranasal sinuses are present at birth. They tend to enlarge rapidly in late childhood and at puberty as the facial bones grow anteriorly and inferiorly from the skull base. In humans, the paranasal sinuses have no known function.

12.2 Clinical examination

Clinical features

Obstruction
This is the most common problem and may be unilat-

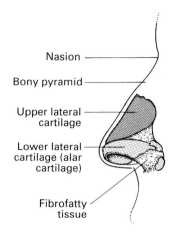

Fig. 109
The external nose.

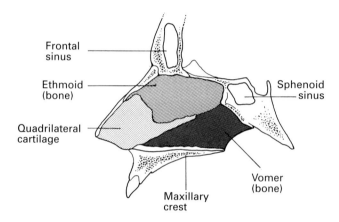

Fig. 110
The nasal septum.

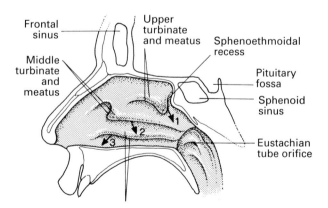

Fig. 111
Structure of the lateral wall of the nasal cavity, showing the upper (1), middle (2), and lower (3) turbinates.

eral or bilateral. The cause may be structural or related to mucosal swelling. Common causes of nasal obstruction include deviation of the nasal septum, mucosal inflammation (rhinitis), nasal polyps and, more rarely, neoplasia.

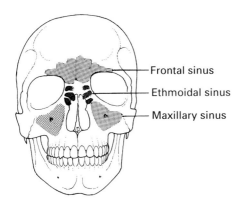

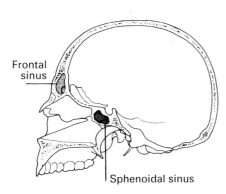

Fig. 112
The paranasal sinuses.

Discharge

This may be clear or coloured, unilateral or bilateral, anterior or posterior (catarrh). Unilateral bloodstained nasal discharge suggests a foreign body in a toddler or a neoplasm in the elderly.

Sneezing

This results from nasal mucosal irritation and is a common feature of allergic rhinitis.

Pain

Facial discomfort and pain may be secondary to sinus obstruction and inflammation.

Anosmia

Anosmia is commonly secondary to nasal obstruction. In the absence of nasal obstruction, alteration of smell may result from disease in the anterior cranial fossa.

Cosmesis

Cosmetic nasal deformities are common and include humps, sagging of the nasal dorsum and deviation of the nose. Complaints about nasal size are also common. Nasal appearance is often racially determined and complaint thresholds vary from culture to culture. Some patients present with complaints about nasal function when their main concern is cosmetic.

Investigations

The exterior and interior of the nose must be carefully examined in all patients with nasal complaints. The external nose should be examined for deviation, scars and skin abnormalities. Standard anterior rhinoscopy using a nasal speculum allows a very limited assessment of the nasal cavities and this examination is best undertaken nowadays with a rigid or flexible endoscope which allows an assessment of the nasopharynx.

In children, the internal nose can be inspected by tilting the nasal tip with the examiner's thumb: instruments tend to frighten children.

The anterior end of the inferior turbinate is often mistaken for a nasal polyp; gentle probing will elicit discomfort from a turbinate but not from a polyp.

Gentle stimulation of the locally anaesthetised nasal septal mucosa will often allow identification of a bleeding spot in Little's area.

Physical examination may be supplemented by imaging including paranasal sinus X-rays, CT and MRI scanning. Allergy testing by skin prick or RAST (radioallergosorbent test) is helpful in patients suspected of having allergic rhinitis. Mucociliary clearance testing and rhinomanometry are becoming used more routinely.

12.3 Infection and inflammation

Rhinitis

The most common cause of rhinitis is the common cold, caused by viral infection. This condition is characterised by nasal obstruction, nasal discharge and sneezing. It is usually self-limiting within 4 to 5 days but may be complicated by secondary bacterial infection. It is most common in young children who have not yet developed immunity to the causative viral agents. Symptoms tend to be more severe and longer lasting in smokers, who have impaired mucociliary function.

Sinusitis

Acute sinusitis may be a complication of the common cold as ventilation of the paranasal sinuses may be impaired by swollen mucosa and thick secretions. Steam inhalations and local or systemic decongestants produce symptomatic relief. Secondary bacterial infection may be treated with broad-spectrum antibiotics. Occasionally, maxillary sinusitis is associated with infection of the apices of the premolar and molar teeth, which protrude into the sinus cavity. Such infections are commonly caused by anaerobic organisms. Typically acute sinusitis of rhinogenic origin is associated with pain located over the affected sinus, nasal obstruction and sometimes purulent nasal discharge. Medical treatment is by decongestants, analgesics and antibiotics. Occasionally, surgical intervention is required to drain the maxillary or frontal sinuses if pain is severe or complications such as orbital cellulitis or intracranial spread of infection threaten.

If acute sinusitis does not resolve adequately, *chronic* sinusitis may develop with further damage to the mucosal lining of the involved sinuses. Medical treatment to improve sinus drainage and reduce infection may help, but surgical intervention is sometimes necessary. Nowadays this is commonly accomplished by functional endoscopic sinus surgery (FESS), rather than by older operations, which were designed to remove damaged mucosa and to provide large drainage channels from the sinuses to the nasal cavity.

Nasal vestibulitis

Inflammation of the nasal vestibules may be secondary to infected anterior nasal discharge or may result from infection of the hair follicles, usually by *Staphylococcus aureus*. In children, vestibulitis is sometimes associated with a foreign body or more rarely with unilateral choanal atresia. Careful examination of the nose is required. Pus should be sent for culture and sensitivity testing, followed by appropriate antibiotic treatment. Diabetic and immunosuppressed patients are more prone to recurrent infection of the hair follicles in the nasal vestibules (furunculosis).

Atrophic rhinitis

This rare condition appears to be associated with poor hygiene and malnutrition. It is characterised by nasal crusting and often with foetor (ozaena). Medical treatment involves removal of the crusts and application of nasal douches and drops. Surgical treatment to reduce the size of the nasal cavities is sometimes needed.

Allergic and non-specific (vasomotor) rhinitis

Allergic rhinitis may be either seasonal or perennial. In the UK, common seasonal allergens include tree and grass pollen in spring and summer, respectively. Mould spores may cause allergies in the autumn. In North America, ragweed pollen is a potent source of allergic symptoms in the late summer.

Perennial allergic rhinitis commonly results from exposure to animal dander, feathers and the house dust mite. Some patients develop nasal symptoms resulting from ingested allergens such as eggs, milk products and various nuts. Allergic rhinitis is common, affecting up to one in five of the population. It results from a type 1 hypersensitivity reaction in which an IgE and allergen complex binds to mast cells. These cells degranulate, releasing inflammatory mediators including histamine.

The nasal mucosa may also react to non-specific stimuli, such as changes in temperature and humidity, and to stress and hormonal changes such as those occurring at puberty and during pregnancy. This type of non-allergic rhinitis is known as *non-specific* or *vasomotor* rhinitis and is mediated by the autonomic innervation of the nasal mucosa.

In both allergic and non-specific rhinitis, nasal obstruction, clear nasal discharge and bouts of sneezing occur. Nowadays, the mainstay of treatment of both types of rhinitis is the use of steroid nasal sprays. These may be used long term, but after symptom control is established a minimum maintenance dose of the spray should be employed. In allergic rhinitis, topical and systemic antihistamine therapy may help as may topical sodium cromoglycate. Surgery in the form of turbinate reduction may help nasal obstruction but does not benefit other manifestations of allergic and vasomotor rhinitis.

Prolonged use of topical nasal decongestants may itself result in nasal inflammation, producing a condition known as rhinitis medicomentosa. This is treated by stopping the use of the topical decongestant and substituting a steroid nasal spray. Compliance is better if one nostril is treated at a time. Systemic decongestants may also help.

12.4 Nasal septum

Trauma

Injuries to the nose may result in damage to nasal soft tissues, cartilage and bone. Patients presenting with nasal injuries should be assessed for associated damage to the head, neck and facial bones. If a nasal septal haematoma is present, it should be drained, the nose packed to prevent reaccumulation of blood and systemic antibiotics given. If the nasal bones are fractured, the nose should be re-examined after a few days when the bruising and swelling has settled to assess any residual cosmetic deformity. This should be corrected by nasal manipulation within 10 to 14 days of the injury; otherwise the bones will heal and the deformity will require formal correction by rhinoplasty. Septal deviations resulting from injury may require surgical correction. Untreated, a septal haematoma may form an abscess with the risk of intracranial spread of infection. Later resorption of the septal cartilage may cause a saddle nose deformity.

Deviation

This may result from differential nasal growth or from trauma. It may involve bone or cartilage of the septum or both. Cartilaginous septal deviations may result in deviation of the external nose. Asymptomatic septal deformities require no treatment but if there is compromise of function or cosmesis, surgical correction by submucosal resection of the septum or by septoplasty is indicated.

Perforation

Perforations are commonly asymptomatic and are seen as an incidental finding. If symptomatic they may produce bleeding, crusting and whistling. They usually result from trauma, often surgical, but may be caused by nose picking and cocaine abuse. Rare infections such as tuberculosis or syphilis may result in septal perforation.

If asymptomatic, perforations require no treatment. Small to medium-sized perforations can be closed surgically or more simply by the placement of a silastic obturator. Large septal perforations may not be amenable to any form of therapy.

12.5 **Epistaxis**

Nose bleeds usually result from disruption of blood vessels in the anterior portion of the septum (Little's area). This area is the site of a rich vascular anastomosis and is relatively easily traumatised. Bleeding is readily controlled by sitting the patient up with the head slightly forward and pinching the tip of the nose. Blood loss from such bleeding is usually not severe. Cautery of the bleeding area can be carried out under local anaesthesia using silver nitrate sticks or electrocautery.

Potentially more serious nose bleeding results from rupture of larger unsupported posteriorly placed vessels. This type of nose bleed tends to occur in elderly patients who are hypertensive and have arterial disease. Blood loss may be extremely rapid and the patient must be assessed clinically for shock. Blood loss in this situation is often underestimated as the patient swallows a great deal of blood. Measurement of pulse and blood pressure is essential and intravenous infusion and blood transfusion are often necessary. The exact site of a posterior nose bleed is often difficult to determine even with adequate illumination and suction. If a bleeding point can be identified with a nasal endoscope, it may be cauterised under endoscopic control. Most such bleeding is controlled by anteriorly placed nasal packing, but occasionally postnasal packing is required. The latter usually requires general anaesthesia. Compressive balloons are available to control bleeding and in an emergency a Foley catheter may be used as a posterior pack. If anterior packing is to be in place for more than 48 hours, systemic antibiotics should be given. The presence of a posterior pack mandates the use of antibiotics.

Underlying causes of severe or continuous bleeding should be sought. Coagulation disorders and patients on anticoagulant therapy may present with severe nose bleeds. Associated conditions such as hypertension need to be controlled. If conservative measures do not control the bleeding, arterial ligation may be necessary. Vessels commonly ligated are the anterior ethmoid and maxillary arteries or occasionally the external carotid artery.

12.6 **Nasal obstruction**

Choanal atresia

Choanal atresia results from failure of breakdown of the bucco-nasal membrane. If bilateral it presents as an acute respiratory obstruction in the neonate, as neonates are obligate nasal breathers. Unilateral cases present later in infancy or childhood with unilateral purulent nasal discharge and obstruction.

Diagnosis

Diagnosis is confirmed by failure to pass a soft catheter through the nostril and can be definitively imaged by CT scanning, which helps to differentiate bony from membranous atresia.

Management

Bilateral atresia in neonates requires establishment of an oral airway as an emergency followed by urgent surgical correction of the atresia. Surgery may be delayed in unilateral cases.

Polyps

Nasal polyps are made up of redundant oedematous mucosa and usually arise from the ethmoid sinuses. Most commonly they are bilateral and present in the middle meatus causing nasal obstruction. Occasionally they arise from the maxillary sinus in which case they pass posteriorly and are known as antrochoanal polyps. They are often associated with infective rhinitis and nasal allergies but do not occur in children except in association with cystic fibrosis. Typically polyps have the appearance of skinned green grapes and are insensitive to probing, unlike inferior turbinates for which they are often mistaken.

Unilateral nasal polyps should be regarded with suspicion. In infants, a polypoid nasal mass may be a congenital abnormality such as a meningoencephalocoele. In adults, unilateral polyps may result from neoplastic growth.

Large polyps require surgical removal possibly with surgery to the associated sinus. Small polyps may be managed by use of local steroid sprays.

Foreign bodies

These are usually seen in toddlers and occasionally in mentally disturbed patients. Inert foreign bodies such as small pebbles or metal ball-bearings may produce few symptoms. Other materials such as foam, wool or vegetable matter result in a brisk inflammatory reaction which produces a purulent, often blood-stained, nasal discharge. This can result in vestibulitis of the ipsilateral nasal skin.

Unless the foreign body can be easily and safely

removed, referral to a rhinologist is indicated. Inhalation of the foreign body during manipulation is a risk and in young children general anaesthesia is sometimes required.

Rhinoliths result from accumulation of calcium and magnesium salts around a foreign body. They may reach a very large size and produce obstruction and discharge. General anaesthesia is often required for their removal.

Self-assessment: questions

Multiple choice questions

1. Causes of recurrent maxillary sinusitis include:
   a. Apical dental infections
   b. Repeated epistaxes
   c. Recurrent bouts of otitis media
   d. Deviation of the nasal septum
   e. Nasal foreign body

2. Epistaxis:
   a. Rarely occurs in children
   b. Most commonly results from rupture of posterior placed nasal vessels
   c. May be treated by ligation of the ipsilateral internal carotid artery
   d. May be treated by cautery of Little's area by silver nitrate
   e. Is the most common cause of emergency admission to ENT wards

3. Allergic rhinitis:
   a. Is caused by a type 1 hypersensitivity reaction
   b. Is best treated by turbinate surgery
   c. Is commonly complicated by profuse nose bleeds
   d. Increases the risk of development of nasal carcinoma
   e. Produces symptoms mainly in elderly people

Case history

A 75-year-old previously healthy man presents to the Accident and Emergency Department with a profuse left-sided nose bleed of sudden onset. He estimates that he has soaked two medium-sized towels with blood and has swallowed a considerable quantity.

1. What are the priorities in the management of this patient?
2. What local measures should be taken to attempt to control the bleeding?
3. What alternative treatments are there?

An anterior nasal pack is placed and he is admitted to hospital. Over the next 48 hours blood continues to trickle through the packing and blood can be seen trickling down the posterior oropharyngeal wall from time

4. What further steps should be taken at this point?
5. How would it be established whether the patient has a generalised bleeding disorder?

6. Assuming further management does not control the bleeding, what further steps can be undertaken?

Picture question

This patient (Fig. 113) has recently sustained a nasal injury, having been struck in the face with an iron bar.

1. What can be done to rule out other injuries?
2. Assuming the nasal bones are fractured, is it necessary to reduce the fracture? How is this decision made?
3. For what period is it possible to undertake a closed reduction of the fracture?
4. If reduction is delayed, what definitive treatment will be required?

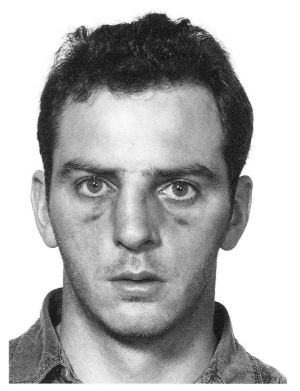

Fig. 113
Patient with a recent nasal fracture.

Short notes

Write short notes on the following:

1. deviated nasal septum
2. allergic rhinitis
3. acute maxillary sinusitis
4. foreign body in the nose.

Self-assessment: answers

Multiple choice answers

1. a. **True.** Apical dental infections are usually caused by anaerobic organisms and the roots of the premolar and molar teeth may project into the antrum with minimal or absent bony covering.
   b. **False.** Epistaxis may be a feature of recurrent maxillary sinusitis, but it is not a cause.
   c. **False.** Otitis media, particularly in children, may be associated with sinus infections, but it is not causative.
   d. **True.** Deviations of the nasal septum may be sufficiently severe to cause impaired drainage of the maxillary sinus, resulting in recurrent infections.
   e. **True.** Nasal foreign bodies are most common in children and the mentally retarded and may result in obstruction of the maxillary sinus ostium producing chronic recurrent infections.

2. a. **False.** Bleeding from Little's area frequently occurs in children and may be associated with nasal vestibulitis.
   b. **False.** Most bleeding results from rupture of vessels in the anterior part of the nasal septum (Little's area).
   c. **False.** If not controlled by cautery and packing, ligation of the external or maxillary artery is appropriate. Ligation of the internal carotid artery could result in stroke or death.
   d. **True.** This is the definitive treatment for most nose bleeds.
   e. **True.** Most such admissions occur in elderly patients in the winter months.

3. a. **True.** This results in degranulation of mass cells with release of histamine and other chemical mediators, which result in the classic symptoms of allergic rhinitis.
   b. **False.** The most appropriate treatment is avoidance of the allergen if possible. Topical nasal steroid sprays are the mainstay of treatment nowadays. Turbinate surgery should be limited to those patients in whom there is an irreversible turbinate hypertrophy.
   c. **False.** Mucosa tends to be swollen by oedema rather than by engorgement with blood.
   d. **False.** There is no association between allergic rhinitis and the development of nasal carcinoma.
   e. **False.** Allergic rhinitis tends to be less troublesome in the elderly. Symptoms tend to be maximal in the teens and twenties.

Case history answer

1. The priorities in management are the same as in any patient who has sustained a significant blood loss. Regular monitoring of blood pressure and pulse are mandatory and if there is actual or impending hypovolaemic shock, attention must be directed to this immediately.
2. An assessment should be made to identify the site of bleeding. This requires a good light source and adequate suction. In epistaxis in the elderly, the source of haemorrhage is usually rupture of a posteriorly placed vessel and packing of the nose with cotton wool wrung out in a local anaesthetic/vasoconstrictor solution will allow a more definitive anterior nasal pack of ribbon gauze smeared with an antibiotic ointment or bismuth iodoform paraffin paste (BIPP) to be placed. Sedation is often helpful, but respiratory depression must be avoided. Nowadays nasal tampons are available commercially and are easier to insert and remove. Endoscopic techniques may also be used to control bleeding by cautery.
3. If anterior packing fails to control the bleeding a posterior pack should be placed. With the use of endonasal telescopes, it is now possible to identify and cauterise individual bleeding points provided the bleeding is not too profuse.
4. An estimate of the blood loss should be made. The history is helpful here. Initial evaluation of the haemoglobin level and haematocrit is not helpful until haemodilution has occurred. Blood transfusion may be necessary. It may be necessary to place a posterior nasal pack in the form of a proprietary balloon or a pre-made pack.
5. A history of previous bleeding tendencies is important. In elderly patients, it is necessary to exclude concomitant therapy with anticoagulants prescribed for thrombo-embolic disease. If in doubt a coagulation screen should be requested.
6. If the measures taken so far do not control the bleeding, arterial ligation should be considered. The most appropriate arteries to ligate are the maxillary artery, access to which is gained via the maxillary antrum, and the anterior ethmoidal artery. The external carotid artery in the neck may be ligated but is further away from the bleeding site with greater risk of continued bleeding via anastomotic vessels.

Picture answer

1. A history of the nature of the injury should be obtained. Significant head and cervical spine injury must be excluded as a priority. The most likely

associated injuries are those to the maxilla or zygoma. Problems with dental occlusion and a palpable step in the inferior orbital rim are features of fracture of the maxilla. Loss of sensation over the cheek suggests damage to the infraorbital nerve which is a feature of an orbital blow-out fracture.

2. The reasons for reducing any facial fracture are to achieve restoration of function and/or to improve cosmesis. If there is no significant deformity and the patient is able to breathe comfortably through both nostrils reduction is not necessary.

3. Reduction should be undertaken within 2 weeks of the time of injury. Up until 10 days, fractured nasal bones are easily manipulated, but after this the nasal bones are much less mobile. Patients with nasal fractures often have had previous injury and the surgeon should obtain information regarding the immediate preinjury appearance prior to undertaking nasal fracture reduction.

4. If reduction is delayed, definitive treatment usually involving a formal rhinoplasty with osteotomies is indicated to restore cosmesis and function.

Short notes answers

1. Deviation of the nasal septum most commonly results from injury. In children and adolescents deviations may become more marked with growth. The condition may cause no symptoms and may be found incidentally at examination. Nasal septal deviation is a common cause of nasal obstruction which may be unilateral or bilateral. It may contribute to recurrent sinus infection because of compromise to aeration and drainage of the sinuses. The caudal end of the septum is commonly dislocated into the nasal vestibule, while further back the septal cartilage lies obliquely producing obstruction on the opposite side. If symptoms are severe surgery in the form of submucosal resection of septal cartilage or nasal septoplasty is indicated.

2. Allergic rhinitis results from IgE binding to mast cells in the nasal mucosa with release of vasoactive agents. Common allergens include grass and tree pollens, mould spores, animal dander and house dust mite faeces. The condition is characterised by clear nasal discharge, sneezing, nasal congestion and conjunctivitis. A detailed history will often indicate the offending allergen and this may be supplemented by skin prick and RAST (Radio Allergo Sorbent Test) blood tests. Avoidance of the offending allergen is the best treatment. Frequently this is very difficult or impossible. Topically applied steroid nasal sprays are extremely effective. Antihistamines are also beneficial. Topical decongestants and systemic steroids may be indicated for short term use. Desensitisation is no longer commonly practised in the United Kingdom.

3. Acute maxillary sinusitis commonly presents following an upper respiratory infection. Rarely it may result from a dental abscess involving a molar or pre-molar tooth or occasionally occurs after a dental extraction. Factors causing impairment of drainage such as nasal polyps or deviation of the nasal septum may be contributory. The condition is characterised by cheek pain which is aggravated by coughing, head movement and walking. Causitive organisms are usually Haemophilus influenzae, Pneumococcus or Staphylococcus. When secondary to dental infection, anaerobic organisms are usually involved. Swelling of the cheek is rare. Medical treatment with appropriate antibiotics, nasal vasoconstrictor drops and analgesics is usually curative.

4. Foreign bodies in the nose most commonly occur in toddlers who place beads, pieces of paper, peanuts, etc. in their noses. The child usually presents with a unilateral foul smelling, occasionally bloodstained discharge with excoriation of the skin of the nasal vestibule. The child will rarely admit to placing a foreign body in the nose and several weeks normally elapse prior to presentation. Removal of the foreign body may be achieved in the cooperative child using local analgesia with appropriate lighting and forceps. In an uncooperative child general anaesthesia will be required.

The throat

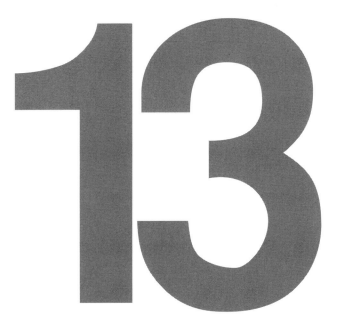

13.1 **Introduction**

Common symptoms are:

- sore throat
- difficulty in swallowing
- changes in the voice
- airway obstruction.

13.2 **Sore throats**

Pharyngitis

Throat infections are usually caused by viral infections and are associated with other upper respiratory tract symptoms. Bacterial infection, commonly streptococcal, may be primary or secondary. Infected sore throats should be treated with oral analgesics, plentiful oral fluids and, if severe, bed rest. Antibiotics are given only if bacterial infection is suspected. Other types of infection include *Candida* spp., which may occur in diabetic or immunocompromised patients and is sometimes seen in patients who use steroid inhalers for asthma. It presents as fluffy white patches on the fauces and responds to topical antifungal agents.

Tonsillitis

Bacterial tonsillitis is characterised by:

- sore throat lasting for a week
- dysphagia (difficulty swallowing)
- odynophagia (pain on swallowing)
- fever
- cervical lymphadenopathy
- malaise.

If recurrent attacks significantly interfere with school or work, tonsillectomy should be considered. Tonsillectomy is generally not indicated for less than three or four attacks of tonsillitis per year.

Complications of tonsillectomy

- reactionary haemorrhage occurs in the first 24 hours following tonsillectomy.
- Secondary haemorrhage occurs a week or so following surgery and is associated with separation of slough from the tonsillar bed.

13.3 **Disorders of swallowing**

Dysphagia is difficulty in swallowing. Odynophagia is pain on swallowing.

Clinical features

Organic dysphagia may arise acutely from foreign body impaction, but this history may be difficult to elicit from young children. More characteristically, dysphagia presents as a progression of difficulty in swallowing solids to difficulty with semisolids and then to difficulty swallowing liquids. It is usually associated with weight loss. If associated with hoarseness, cervical lymphadenopathy and otalgia cancer should be suspected. Dysphagia associated with aspiration of liquids suggests neuromuscular disease. The sensation of a lump in the throat without dysphagia is termed globus pharyngis. The need to swallow twice, particularly if associated with regurgitation of undigested food following a meal, suggests a pharyngeal pouch.

Diagnosis

A limited examination of the hypopharynx can be undertaken using the laryngeal mirror or fibreoptic endoscope. A barium swallow will usually define a lower lesion.

Classification

- Intrinsic lesions, e.g. neoplasia, diverticulum, stricture, achalasia.
- Extrinsic lesions, e.g. goitre, mediastinal masses.
- Generalised disease, e.g. scleroderma, dermatomyositis.
- Neuromuscular disorders, e.g. myasthenia gravis, motor neurone disease, disseminated sclerosis.

13.4 **Change in the voice**

Hoarseness or dysphonia is an alteration in the quality of the voice. Aphonia is absence of voice. The most common cause is acute laryngitis associated with viral infection and is self-limiting. The inflammation is exacerbated by smoking, alcohol and voice abuse. If these factors are not corrected, chronic laryngitis may develop.

Voice abuse may lead to nodules (singer's or screamer's nodules) at the junction of the anterior third and posterior two-thirds of the true vocal cord. It may also result in polypoid changes in the vocal cords and frank polyps may form. Speech therapy is essential to correct poor vocal habits. Surgical removal is indicated for lesions that do not resolve with conservative therapy. Hoarseness may result from neoplastic disease of the larynx and hoarseness persisting for more than 3 weeks should be investigated by indirect laryngoscopy.

The voice quality in unilateral vocal cord palsy is variable depending on the position of the paralysed cord in relation to its mobile partner. If there is a significant gap between the vocal cords on phonation, the voice is weak and breathy. The patient may also have difficulty with aspiration of liquids. In bilateral cord palsy, the voice may be good, but the airway is often inadequate. Vocal cord palsy may be idiopathic or result from damage to the laryngeal nerve supply anywhere between the brain stem and the mediastinum.

13.5 **Airway obstruction**

Stertor is the name given to the sound resulting from obstruction of the airway above the larynx. The sound is characterised by a snuffling, snorting quality. Snoring results from vibration of the tissues of the soft palate and pharynx. Complete or partial airway obstruction during snoring may result from collapse of the hypopharyngeal airway and also from posterior displacement of the base of the tongue. During sleep the airway may become periodically completely obstructed causing sleep apnoea. In young children in whom the tonsils may be relatively large and the pharynx relatively small this is a recognised cause of sleep apnoea which is an indication for tonsillectomy in the young child. In older children and young adults infectious mononucleosis may result in marked tonsillar hypertrophy, again with the risk of airway obstruction. Tumours of the tongue base and pharynx rarely become large enough to produce airway obstruction — dysphagia is a more common presenting feature.

Airway obstruction resulting from laryngeal disease may present at any age. Congenital abnormalities of the larynx may result in stridor at birth. Laryngomalacia, a condition in which the laryngeal cartilages are soft and floppy, is a common cause of stridor in the first year of life. Acute supraglottitis (epiglottitis) results from H. influenza infection and presents with airway obstruction and drooling in the young child. The onset is rapid and the child sits in an upright position struggling for breath. This is an acute emergency. The child requires immediate transfer to hospital where the airway is usually established by passage of a nasotracheal tube in a setting where facilities for bronchoscopy and tracheostomy are available.

Bilateral paralysis of the vocal cords is a rarer cause of airway obstruction at all ages. Carcinoma of the larynx occasionally presents as airway obstruction. This is particularly true where the tumour involves the supraglottis or subglottis. Such patients are occasionally misdiagnosed as having asthma. The noisy breathing in this condition is stridor not wheeze!

13.6 **Clinical examination**

With a good source of illumination, tongue depressors, gauze swabs (to gently draw the tongue forwards) and appropriate mirrors, the entire oral cavity, pharynx and larynx can be examined. Mucosal surfaces should be carefully inspected and if necessary palpated. Palpation is particularly important in assessing oral cavity lesions. Fibre-optic telescopes, both rigid and flexible, may be necessary to examine those patients in whom mirrors do not give an adequate view. Examination of the neck includes inspection and palpation in a systematic fashion. The entire neck should be exposed which may necessitate the removal of high necked shirts.

Imaging techniques, including plain and contrast radiology, CT and MR scanning are useful adjuncts to physical examination.

Self-assessment: questions

Multiple choice questions

1. Complications of tonsillectomy include:
   a. Secondary haemorrhage
   b. Severe otalgia
   c. Quinsy
   d. Nasopharyngeal stenosis
   e. Intracranial abscess

2. Hypopharyngeal diverticulum:
   a. Is associated with achalasia of the oesophagus
   b. Is a premalignant condition
   c. Is uncommon in people over age 50 years
   d. Tends to regress with time
   e. Is associated with iron-deficiency anaemia

3. Features characteristic of acute tonsillitis include:
   a. Sublingual swelling
   b. Odynophagia
   c. Croupy cough
   d. Referred otalgia
   e. Haemoptysis

4. A 6-month-old baby has had mild inspiratory stridor for the last 2 months. Possible causes include:
   a. Subglottic stenosis
   b. Acute epiglottitis
   c. Croup

d. Tonsillar hypertrophy
e. Laryngomalacia

Case history

> An 85-year-old female patient with increasing dysphagia of 8 months' duration feels generally lethargic and has lost 10 lb in weight over the last few months. Clinical examination of the head and neck reveals no abnormalities.

1. What investigations should be requested?
2. Barium swallow shows a postcricoid web; what should be done next?
3. Will correcting the anaemia make the web disappear?
4. What condition is associated with postcricoid web?
5. How should this condition be treated?

Short notes

Write short notes on:

1. the indications for tonsillectomy
2. the investigation of dysphagia in the elderly
3. causes of hoarseness in the young adult
4. treatment of chronic laryngitis
5. aetiology of vocal cord paralysis

Self-assessment: answers

Multiple choice answers

1. a. **True.** Secondary haemorrhage may occur between the fifth and tenth day postoperatively. The bleeding is not usually as severe as that in primary haemorrhage and appears to be associated with infection of the tonsillar bed during separation of the fibrinous slough.
    b. **True.** Severe otalgia, mediated by the glossopharyngeal nerve, may occur in the first week to 10 days following tonsillectomy.
    c. **False.** Quinsy, by definition, is a peritonsillar abscess and cannot occur after the tonsil has been removed.
    d. **True.** This may result from excessive removal of palatal mucosa. The palate subsequently heals by scarring, resulting in narrowing of the nasopharynx.
    e. **False.** Localised infection of the tonsillar bed may occur. More generalised infection is extremely rare.

2. a. **False.** The two conditions are quite distinct.
    b. **False.** Malignancy in hypopharyngeal diverticulum has been reported only extremely rarely.
    c. **False.** This disease tends to occur in people over the age of 50.
    d. **False.** The diverticulum tends to enlarge with time.
    e. **False.** The Plummer–Vinson syndrome, not hypopharyngeal diverticulum, is classically associated with iron-deficiency anaemia.

3. a. **False.** Some swelling of the soft palate may be seen. Swelling under the tongue is not a feature of acute tonsillitis.
    b. **True.** The fauces are inflamed and swallowing is painful.
    c. **False.** Cough is not a feature of acute tonsillitis.
    d. **True.** Ear pain referred via the glossopharyngeal nerve is not uncommon in acute tonsillitis.
    e. **False.** Haemoptysis is not a feature of acute tonsillitis.

4. a. **True.** Subglottic narrowing may be congenital or acquired. Acquired cases usually result from prolonged endotracheal intubation. Most congenital cases are self limiting as the child grows.
    b. **False.** Acute epiglottitis develops rapidly, usually in a period of hours. It would not cause symptoms for 2 months.
    c. **False.** Acute laryngotracheo-bronchitis develops rapidly and is associated with a characteristic cough.
    d. **False.** Tonsillar hypertrophy may cause airway obstruction producing stertor. Stridor results from narrowing of the laryngeal or tracheal airway.
    e. **True.** This is a common cause of stridor in this age group.

Case history answer

1. The most valuable investigation in a patient complaining of progressive dysphagia is a barium swallow. A full blood count would also be appropriate given her history of lethargy.
2. The patient requires endoscopy to exclude associated malignancy. The web on barium swallow is often endoscopically found to be a mucosal fold and may be difficult to identify. Nevertheless, the area requires to be examined directly.
3. In many patients, correcting the anaemia will cause an early web to resolve.
4. Postcricoid carcinoma is the life-threatening condition associated with postcricoid web.
5. Early, limited postcricoid carcinomas may be treated by radical radiotherapy. More extensive tumours require radical surgery, which may involve a total laryngo-pharyngo-oesophagectomy with stomach pull up.

Short notes answers

1. Fewer tonsillectomies are performed in the UK than was the case 10 years ago. The most common indication for tonsillectomy is recurrent tonsillitis involving five to six attacks of acute tonsillitis in a single year or three to four per year in a 2 to 3 year period. Major criteria in arriving at a decision are the severity and duration of the symptoms and the amount of school/work lost per year. Tonsils are rarely large enough to cause airway obstruction but may do so in young children. Carcinoma of the tonsil is an absolute indication for tonsillectomy for biopsy. A single quinsy is not nowadays considered an absolute indication for tonsillectomy.
2. The history of the onset, type and duration of dysphagia in the elderly often gives a clue to the type of disease involved. Lesions such as oesophageal stricture, oesophageal carcinoma, hypopharyngeal diverticulum and postcricoid webs all need to be considered. The most useful single investigation is barium swallow, followed by endoscopy and biopsy.
3. Hoarseness in the young adult is unlikely to be caused by carcinoma, which is the potentially most serious cause of hoarseness. Benign lesions such as nodules, polyps or papillomas are more likely. Vocal cord palsy is unlikely but will often present as a

weak breathy voice associated with aspiration of liquids.

4. Chronic laryngitis may result from infection in the upper or lower aerodigestive tracts and this should be sought out and eliminated. Other causes of chronic laryngeal inflammation include irritation by noxious substances, such as may occur in industrial environments. Vocal abuse in the form of overuse or incorrect use of the voice is a common associated factor in the development of chronic laryngitis. Gastro-oesophageal reflux with spillover of acid into the larynx may result in chronic laryngitis.

5. Vocal cord palsy may result from disease anywhere from the brain stem to the mediastinum. Because of its longer course in the thorax, the left recurrent laryngeal nerve is more vulnerable. Intrathoracic disease, such as mediastinal lymphadenopathy and aortic aneurysm, may result in left vocal cord palsy. In the neck, malignant disease, particularly of the thyroid gland and occasionally in the larynx itself, may result in cord palsy. Brain stem disease such as infarct or tumour is usually associated with other neurological features.

Head and neck neoplasia

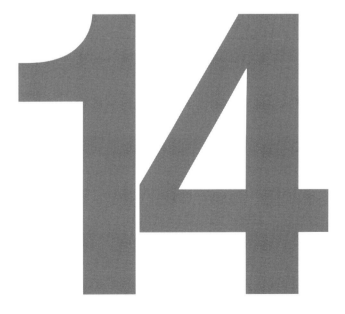

14.1 **Clinical examination**

Presentation

Most malignant tumours of the mucosal surfaces of the head and neck are squamous cell carcinomas. Adenocarcinomas and lymphomas are less common. Squamous cell carcinomas spread by metastasising locally to the regional cervical lymph nodes. These tumours may disrupt breathing, swallowing and speech, are often painful and may alter the patient's appearance. Most squamous cell carcinomas of the mucosal surfaces of the head and neck in western countries are associated with tobacco and alcohol abuse. In the Indian subcontinent betel nut chewing is a predisposing factor. The Epstein–Barr virus has been implicated in the development of nasopharyngeal carcinoma and Burkitt's lymphoma and may possibly predispose to other head and neck cancers too. Exposure to radiation may result in the development of malignancy many years later. Premalignant conditions include leucoplakia (white mucosal patches), erythroplakia (red mucosal patches) and erosive lichen planus.

Diagnosis

In the clinical examination the oral cavity should be examined in a systematic fashion, with careful inspection of the floor and roof of the mouth. When a laryngeal mirror is used, the tongue is pulled very gently to avoid pressure on the undersurface of the tongue from the lower teeth.

A flexible rhinolaryngoscope allows ready examination of the nasopharynx, larynx and hypopharynx.

The regions of the neck are examined in a systematic fashion. To palpate the deep cervical lymph nodes, place the examining fingers deep to the anterior border of the sterno-mastoid muscle: warn the patient that this may be slightly uncomfortable.

The clinical examination is supported by endoscopy and biopsy.

Management

Most squamous cell cancers of the head and neck are treated primarily by surgery, radiation or a combination of both. Chemotherapy is best used in the context of controlled clinical trials. Occasionally, patients present with such advanced disease that no curative treatment is possible. Such patients require physical and psychological support, often best provided in hospice care.

14.2 **The larynx**

It is important to distinguish between stridor, which arises from large airway obstruction, and wheeze, which originates in the smaller airways. Stertor is the term used to denote noisy breathing resulting from partial airway obstruction above the larynx.

Benign tumours

These are best treated with a carbon dioxide laser. Multiple treatments may be required.

Malignant tumours

Squamous cell carcinoma of the larynx most commonly affects the glottis (vocal cords) and presents with hoarseness. Any patient whose hoarseness persists for more than 3 weeks should be examined by indirect laryngoscopy. Early glottic disease has a good prognosis. The true vocal cords have no lymphatic drainage and 95% of patients with squamous cell carcinoma limited to the glottis can, therefore, be cured by radical radiotherapy. Cancers involving the area of the larynx above the vocal cords (supraglottis) and below the vocal cords (subglottis) have a much poorer prognosis as they present later and spread to cervical lymph nodes is more common because of the rich lymphatic drainage from these areas. Patients with very large tumours may present with stridor and dysphagia. Such patients may require urgent tracheostomy prior to definitive therapy.

Management

A few patients with laryngeal carcinoma may be suitable for partial laryngectomy; but in the UK most laryngeal cancers are treated with radical radiotherapy. Once a radical course of radiotherapy has been completed, further radiotherapy cannot be given because of the risk of damage to normal issue.

Total laryngectomy is reserved for patients with very large tumours at presentation and those who fail to respond to radiotherapy. Total laryngectomy involves the creation of an end tracheostome, which is brought out to the surface of the skin. The pharyngeal mucosa is reconstituted over a nasogastric tube and healing occurs in non-radiated patients within 7 to 10 days. Healing takes about twice as long in patients who have previously undergone radiotherapy.

Following total laryngectomy, about one in five patients develops oesophageal speech, which involves vibration of a segment of the reconstituted pharynx and upper oesophagus by swallowed air. Alternative methods include various hand-held battery-powered devices that are held against the neck skin and produce vibration in the pharyngo-oesophageal segment.

14.3 **The oral cavity**

Most malignancies are squamous cell carcinomas and the prognosis tends to be worse the further back in the mouth the tumour is sited. Neoplasms presenting anteriorly in the oral cavity are readily seen whereas those more posteriorly placed often grow large producing relatively few symptoms and metastasise early to the cervical lymph nodes. As well as tobacco and alcohol exposure, poor dental hygiene and teeth with sharp irregular edges are thought to promote malignant change in the oral epithelium. In the Indian subcontinent, betel nut quid which contains tobacco is an important causative factor.

Squamous carcinomas of the lip are usually treated by surgical excision. They present early and usually have a good prognosis.

Carcinoma of the tongue usually presents as an ulcerated lesion on the lateral border. The ulcer is initially painless, but when superinfection and deeper invasion occur, pain is experienced either locally or referred to the ipsilateral ear. Tumours arising in the posterior third of the tongue and in the area of the retromolar trigone (posterior to the third molar tooth) often present late with cervical metastases, so the prognosis is poorer.

Management

Small malignancies of the oral cavity do well with either surgery or radiotherapy. Larger tumours do poorly no matter what modality of treatment is employed. With improved reconstructive techniques, large oral cavity defects can be closed providing adequate rehabilitation of speech and swallowing. Free radial forearm flaps and pectoralis major myocutaneous flaps are routinely used in this type of reconstruction. If the mandible is involved by tumour, to a limited degree marginal mandibulectomy may be possible, preserving the integrity of the mandibular arch. If full thickness bone of the mandible is removed, this can be replaced by bone from the radius in association with a forearm flap.

Carcinoma of the buccal mucosa, often associated with pipe smoking, may be treated by vaporisation using a carbon dioxide laser. An alternative approach uses excision of the mucosa in association with a split skin grafting. Metastatic cervical lymph node disease is usually managed by neck dissection, but small nodes may respond to radiotherapy. When surgery is performed, the primary tumour and the neck dissection specimen are removed in continuity.

14.4 **The pharynx**

Oropharynx

The oropharynx and hypopharynx have a rich lymphatic supply and squamous cell cancers in these areas commonly present with cervical lymphadenopathy. Tumours in this area have a large space in which to grow before symptoms are apparent. Referred otalgia may be a presenting complaint. Patients with tumours in this area often have a high alcohol intake and are heavy smokers who often take little care of themselves. The extent of disease is assessed (usually under general

anaesthesia), by inspection and palpation. Imaging with MRI and CT is helpful in determining the exact extent of tissue involvement.

Management

Treatment involves surgery, radiotherapy or a combination of both. Following surgery reconstruction is by local or distant flaps.

Hypopharyngeal tumours may require laryngopharyngectomy with or without oesophagectomy, and reconstruction is by an interposed viscus, such as stomach, colon or jejunum.

The oropharynx is the most common site of presentation of extranodal lymphoma. These are usually non-Hodgkin's lymphomas and present as mass lesions usually in the area of the tonsil. Staging studies need to be undertaken. If localised, they respond to radiotherapy.

Nasopharynx

Benign tumours

Angiofibroma of the nasopharynx is a rare tumour that typically presents in adolescent males with nasal obstruction and epistaxis. Although histologically benign, they are often locally aggressive, extending laterally into the infratemporal fossa and occasionally through the skull base to the intracranial cavity.

CT, MRI and angiography are all used to define the extent of tumour.

They are usually removed surgically, sometimes with immediate preoperative embolisation to reduce vascularity. For those lesions that cannot be surgically removed safely, radiation is an alternative treatment.

Malignant tumours

Carcinoma of the nasopharynx has its highest incidence in south-east Asia, particularly in the Chinese population of Hong Kong. The Epstein–Barr virus has been implicated in the development of this tumour. The viral genome is incorporated into the DNA of the normal cell, which may become malignant in response to other environmental agents. Because the tumour has a large space in which to grow undetected, presentation is late and variable.

Clinical features

- cervical lymphadenopathy
- otitis media with effusion (indicating obstruction of the Eustachian tube)
- facial pain and altered facial sensation (indicating fifth nerve involvement)
- Horner's syndrome (indicating invasion of the sympathetic chain).

Diagnosis. Diagnosis is made by examination and biopsy. Submucosal lesions can be difficult to detect clinically and may even be missed by biopsy. The extent of the tumour is defined by CT or MRI scanning. Epstein–Barr virus antibody titres may be used to follow the response to treatment and to detect recurrence of disease.

Management. These tumours are treated by radiotherapy. The prognosis is poor, only about one-third of patients surviving for 5 years.

14.5 The nose and paranasal sinuses

Benign tumours

Benign tumours are:

- osteoma
- papilloma: squamous or transitional cell.

Squamous papillomas are common in the nasal vestibule and are treated with cautery or excision. Inverting papilloma, although histologically benign, behaves aggressively and requires extensive removal of the lateral nasal wall. About 10% of inverting papillomas are associated with squamous cell carcinoma.

Osteomas of the fronto-ethmoid complex often present with symptoms of obstruction of the fronto-nasal duct. They are slow growing but if symptomatic require removal.

Malignant tumours

Malignant tumours include:

- squamous cell carcinoma (most common)
- adenocarcinoma
- transitional cell carcinoma
- amaplastic tumours and lymphoma
- olfactory aesthesioneuroblastoma
- minor salivary gland tumour
- melanoma.

Wegener's granuloma is a systemic disease associated with necrotising granulation of the nose. Death is usually caused by associated renal disease.

Lethal mid-line granuloma is a T cell lymphoma and is treated by radiotherapy.

Clinical features

The maxillary sinus is most commonly involved in malignancy. The patient presents with features resulting from the tumour breaching the walls of the antrum. Diplopia indicates orbital involvement; ill-fitting teeth or dentures indicate extension to the oral cavity. Nasal obstruction results from a breach of the medial wall of the antrum. A bleeding polyp in an elderly patient should be regarded with suspicion.

Diagnosis

The extent of disease is defined by CT scanning and a tissue diagnosis obtained by biopsy.

Management

Treatment involves radical radiotherapy followed by surgery. Functional and cosmetic rehabilitation is usually provided by prostheses. The prognosis is poor with a 66% mortality by 5 years.

14.6 The salivary glands

Of all salivary gland neoplasms, 80% occur in the parotid and of these 80–90% are benign. Generally speaking, however, the smaller the salivary gland the more likely it is that a tumour involving the gland will be malignant. In the submandibular gland, about 50% of tumours are malignant and in the minor salivary glands about 90% are malignant.

Benign tumours

- pleomorphic adenoma
- monomorphic adenoma
- Warthin's tumour.

Malignant tumours

- adenoid cystic carcinoma
- squamous cell carcinoma
- pleomorphic carcinoma.

Tumours of intermediate malignancy

- mucoepidermoid tumour
- acinic cell tumour.

Pleomorphic adenoma

This presents as a slowly growing painless lump usually below and little behind the earlobe. It should not be mistaken for an upper cervical lymph node. It does not invade the facial nerve but if present for many years may undergo malignant change.

Fine needle aspiration cytology may help in establishing histological diagnosis.

Treatment is by superficial or total parotidectomy, depending on the part of the gland involved, taking care to preserve the facial nerve.

Warthin's tumour

This parotid tumour usually occurs in older men and is often bilateral. Clinically it feels soft. Histological examination reveals lymphoid tissue.

Malignant tumours

These tend to grow rapidly, invade the facial nerve and are usually painful. Adenoid cystic carcinoma is the most common. This tumour spreads by invasion of the perineural spaces. Local spread is to the cervical lymph nodes and distant spread is commonly to lungs.

CT and MRI scan show the extent of disease.

Treatment involves parotidectomy with facial nerve excision if necessary.

Self-assessment: questions

Multiple choice questions

1. Nasopharyngeal carcinoma:
   a. Is most common in people from south-east China
   b. Presents early with nasal pain
   c. Is treated by wide surgical excision
   d. Is monitored by measurement of Epstein–Barr virus antibodies
   e. Is curable in 90% of patients

2. Carcinoma of the hypopharynx:
   a. Is usually an adenocarcinoma histologically
   b. May present with referred otalgia
   c. Is best treated by chemotherapy
   d. Is often disseminated widely throughout the body at time of presentation
   e. Is curable in 90% of patients

3. In carcinoma of the larynx:
   a. Hoarseness is the most common presenting complaint
   b. Dysphagia is uncommon
   c. Radiation therapy is reserved for inoperable disease
   d. Distant spread to lungs and liver is common
   e. Chemotherapy is the primary modality of treatment

4. Factors which contribute to the development of squamous cell cancers of the head and neck include:
   a. Cigarette smoking
   b. Alcohol ingestion
   c. Ageing
   d. Exposure to particulate emissions from diesel engines
   e. Solar irradiation

Case histories

History 1

> A 55-year-old man attends his GP with hoarseness of 4 weeks' duration following an upper respiratory tract infection. He has no other ENT symptoms. He is in good health and he smokes about 20 cigarettes per day and has done so for the last 40 years.

1. What should the GP do?

> The patient has received radical radiotherapy for an early vocal cord carcinoma. He fails to attend hospital for regular follow-up and 6 months later represents to his GP with a 3-week history of noisy breathing.

2. What is the likely cause of this?
3. What should the GP do?

> Following total laryngectomy, he fails to develop speech.

4. Can anything be done?

> Four months after total laryngectomy he develops a hard lymph node in his neck.

5. What is the most appropriate treatment for this?

History 2

> A 55-year-old man has a slowly enlarging tumour in the right cheek.

1. What is the most likely diagnosis?
2. How could a histological diagnosis be obtained without performing an open biopsy?
3. Is the facial nerve likely to be involved?
4. What is the most appropriate treatment?
5. What complication of therapy should the patient be advised about?

Essay questions

1. Give an account of the therapeutic modalities currently used in the treatment of squamous cell malignancies of the mucosal surfaces of the head and neck.
2. Many head and neck cancers are diagnosed late; why is this?

Self-assessment: answers

Multiple choice answers

1. a. **True.** Nasopharyngeal carcinoma is the most common malignant tumour in men from the Hong Kong area of China.
   b. **False.** Pain is a late feature.
   c. **False.** Radical radiotherapy is the mainstay of treatment.
   d. **True.** Antibodies to specific parts of the Epstein–Barr virus are a sensitive measure of the presence of active tumour.
   e. **False.** Overall survival in all series is much less than 90%.

2. a. **False.** Like most carcinomas of the mucosal surfaces of the head and neck, squamous cell carcinoma is the most common variant.
   b. **True.** Involvement of the superior laryngeal branch of the vagus nerve results in otalgia.
   c. **False.** Surgery and radiotherapy are the mainstays of treatment.
   d. **False.** Early metastases are to the cervical lymph nodes. Widespread dissemination throughout the body is a late feature.
   e. **False.** These tumours are commonly far advanced at the time of presentation and 5-year survival rates are generally less than 50%.

3. a. **True.** Most laryngeal carcinomas arise on the true vocal cord, resulting in alteration of voice quality as the presenting complaint.
   b. **True.** Only very large laryngeal carcinomas impinge on the swallowing passage and dysphagia is usually a late feature.
   c. **False.** Radiation therapy is the mainstay of treatment of all but very advanced laryngeal carcinoma in the UK. Limited tumours of the true vocal cord are cured by radiotherapy in over 90% of patients. The voice is preserved.
   d. **False.** Distant spread is a late feature. In common with most head and neck squamous cell carcinomas, laryngeal cancer spreads initially locally and then to the cervical lymph nodes.
   e. **False.** Chemotherapy should only be used in the context of controlled clinical trials.

4. a. **True.** In western societies this is the major risk factor for the development of squamous cell cancers of the mucosal surfaces of the head and neck. The disease is extremely rare in people who have never smoked.
   b. **True.** Alcohol ingestion is an independent, but less significant risk factor.
   c. **True.** Squamous cell cancers of the head and neck are rarely seen under the age of 50 years.

d. **False.** Diesel fumes are not a recognised aetiological factor.
e. **True.** As far as the skin of the head and neck is concerned solar irradiation is a recognised factor. It is not a risk factor for the development of carcinoma of the mucosal surfaces.

Case history answers

History 1

1. The most important form of management at this stage is to perform an indirect laryngoscopy. Few GPs are equipped or trained to do this. Referral to a laryngologist is, therefore, necessary.
2. Radical radiotherapy is the standard treatment in the UK for early vocal cord carcinoma. Following radiotherapy, patients are usually followed up on a monthly basis either by the laryngologist or at a combined clinic attended by the laryngologist and the radiotherapist. This allows early detection of residual or recurrent tumour. If such follow-up does not occur, residual or recurrent tumour will be missed and may present as airway obstruction, hence this patient's history of noisy breathing.
3. Again the GP is limited in making an appropriate assessment and, therefore, emergency rereferral to the laryngologist is appropriate. Because radical radiotherapy involves a maximum dose of radiotherapy, no further radiotherapy can be given because of damage to the larynx and associated structures. Therefore, laryngectomy is the only remaining therapeutic option.
4. In many centres, a speaking valve is inserted at laryngectomy. Should this not have been done, an assessment should be made by an experienced speech therapist using videofluoroscopy to assess why speech has not developed. Further surgery in the form of a pharyngeal myotomy or valve insertion would most likely be appropriate.
5. Despite the fact that the primary tumour in the larynx has been controlled, cervical lymph nodes containing cancer may present at a later stage. Given that the fields of the original radiotherapy would probably have included the site of the cervical lymph node, neck dissection is the appropriate treatment. In the classical operation, this will involve resection of the internal jugular vein, sternomastoid muscle and accessory nerve.

History 2

1. The mass involves the area of the right parotid salivary gland. Over 80% of tumours in this area are

pleomorphic adenomas. This is compatible with the age of the patient and the fact that the tumour has been slowly enlarging. Other salivary gland tumours are possible, as are tumours in adjacent structures, but pleomorphic adenoma, sometimes known as mixed tumour, of the parotid gland is the most likely mass in this area.

2. Fine needle aspiration cytology (FNAC) is the most appropriate way of obtaining cells for examination from the mass without the need to perform open biopsy.

3. The facial nerve is not likely to be involved by a benign tumour of the parotid gland. Benign tumours grow slowly and the large motor fibres in the nerve can adapt to slowly increasing pressure. This is in contrast to malignant tumours, which invade the nerve early and will result in facial weakness or spasm when the tumour is relatively small.

4. In an otherwise healthy 55-year-old male, superficial parotidectomy is the most appropriate treatment. Such tumours arise most commonly in the superficial lobe of the parotid gland and if left there is a small risk of malignant change; and although they are slowly growing, these tumours can become cosmetically unacceptable.

5. The main risk of superficial parotidectomy is damage to the facial nerve. In skilled surgical hands, this risk is small, but the course of the nerve is variable and the nerve is at risk even in small tumours. To remove the tumour, the great auricular nerve has to be divided and this results in an area of loss of sensation on the side of the face and in the ear-lobe. Some patients postoperatively become aware of sweating from the skin overlying the salivary gland when eating or thinking of food (gustatory sweating). This results from aberrant innervation from nerve fibres that originally supplied the salivary gland tissue regrowing into the sweat glands of the overlying skin. This condition is known as Frey's syndrome.

Essay answers

1. Generally speaking, the therapeutic modalities available for treatment of squamous cell cancers of the mucosal surfaces of the head and neck include surgery and radiotherapy, with chemotherapy being reserved usually for advanced tumours in the context of controlled clinical trials. In early limited tumours, e.g. of the tongue, surgery or radiotherapy are equally effective and the choice often lies as to which modality produces less patient discomfort and most optimally preserves function. For example, early carcinoma of the vocal cord is treated by radiotherapy as this has a minimal effect on the voice.

In more advanced tumours, surgery and radiotherapy are often combined, with surgery preceding radiotherapy in some circumstances and vice versa in others. Some patients present with malignancies at such an advanced stage that cure is not possible and palliative treatment only may be the best option for the patient.

2. Patients who develop squamous cell carcinomas of the mucosal surfaces of head and neck often smoke heavily and abuse alcohol. They tend to be self-neglectful and seek medical treatment late. Tumours in particular areas of the head and neck may grow large before producing symptoms. For example, the nasopharynx and hypopharynx are spaces in which tumours can develop undetected. Many such tumours are not painful in their early stages and symptoms such as hoarseness and dysphagia may be ignored for many months. Patients with head and neck cancers often have other diseases such as chronic bronchitis and cardiovascular disease, which to the patient produce more pressing symptoms than the apparently innocent features of head and neck cancer.

Ophthalmology

Section

3

History taking and examination of the ophthalmic patient

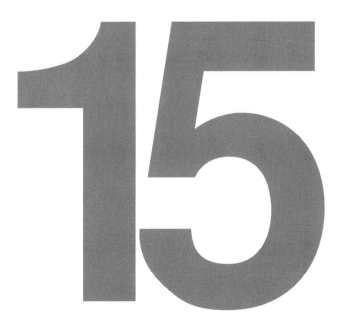

15.1 History

Examination of the patient with an ocular complaint should be carried out in a systematic manner after a clear and accurate history of the problem has been ascertained.

Patients commonly present with symptoms of

- visual loss, which may be gradual, sudden or intermittent or may affect only one part of the visual field
- pain in or around the eyes
- red eyes
- discharge from the eyes.

It is important to determine whether the symptoms affect one or both eyes, the duration, periodicity and severity of symptoms, any relieving or aggravating factors and associated symptoms (e.g. vomiting, headache).

15.2 Examination

Examination should consist of an assessment of

- visual acuity
- external eye
- pupil responses
- ocular motility
- fields of vision.

Visual acuity

Vision is assessed using a standard Snellen chart (Fig. 114A). Each eye is tested in turn, testing the right eye first as routine. If the patient wears glasses, they should be worn for the test, and if the patient is unable to read the chart then they should be asked to look through a pin-hole aperture as this neutralises any refractive error. The chart should be placed 6 metres from the patient, who is asked to read the chart from the top. If they are only able to see the top letter then the acuity is documented as 6/60 (a person with normal vision should be able to see the top letter from 60 metres away). If the chart can be read to the bottom, then the acuity is 6/6, i.e. normal vision. If the patient is unable to see the chart at all, then vision should be recorded progressively as the ability to count fingers (CFs), perceive hand movements (HMs), perceive light (PL) or not perceive light (NPL).

Near vision should also be tested. This can be done using a standard reading book, although if this is not available any text would do.

Children, obviously, cannot read letters and, therefore, there are tests available using pictures (Kay's pictures, Fig. 114B) and individual letters for which they can point to matching letters on a card (Sheridan Gardiner test).

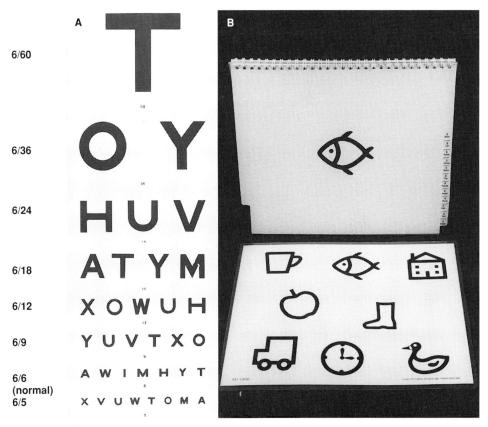

Fig. 114
Methods of testing visual acuity. **A.** The Snellen chart. **B.** Kay's pictures.

The external eye

The eye should be examined using a good light and magnification if possible. Magnification can be obtained using the plus 10 dioptre lens in the ophthalmoscope. The lids, tear film, conjunctiva and sclera (Fig. 115) should be inspected. Loss of the bright corneal reflex is a useful sign of an epithelial abnormality. A drop of fluorescein (1%) should be instilled into the conjunctival sac as this stains areas of epithelial loss bright green when viewed with a blue light. This helps to identify corneal foreign bodies or abrasions. If the patient has any symptoms of foreign body sensation, the upper lid should be everted (Fig. 116). The anterior chamber should be examined to determine its depth and the presence of any blood or pus.

Pupils

The pupils should not be dilated for examination of the retina without first examining the pupil responses.

Check that the pupils are round and equal under ambient lighting.

Examine the pupillary responses to light. Shine a bright light into each eye checking that there is a direct and consensual response in each eye and that these responses are equal. If the direct response is less than the consensual response this indicates an 'afferent pupillary defect' (see Ch. 23 and Fig. 150).

Examine the pupillary responses to accommodation. The reaction to accommodation is tested by asking the patient to look in the distance and then asking them to fix on an object held at approximately 30 cm from their nose. Both pupils should constrict when looking at the near object.

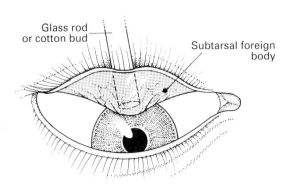

Fig. 116
Everting the upper lid. Ask the patient to look downwards and evert the lid over a glass rod or cotton bud by pulling on the lashes.

Ocular motility

Any patient with a suspected squint should be examined using the cover test and examination of the extraocular movements.

Cover test

This is the basic examination for the patient with a squint (Fig. 117). Only by carrying out this test can one determine whether a patient has a squint or not. Ask the patient to fix on an interesting target held 60–90 cm away. In a non-squinting person, when either eye is covered the other eye does not move. In a person with, for example, a convergent squint then the squinting eye will move from its inturning position in an outwards direction to take up fixation when the other eye is covered. In a divergent squint, the diverging eye moves inwards to take up fixation.

Extraocular eye movements

The eyes must be examined in all nine positions of gaze

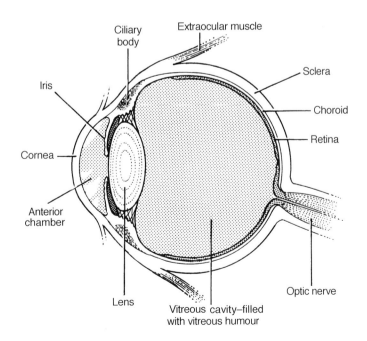

Fig. 115
Anatomy of the eye.

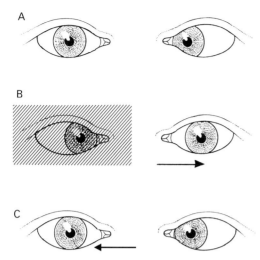

Fig. 117
The cover test. **A.** Patient fixating the target; the left eye appears convergent. **B.** The right eye is covered and the left eye moves out to take up fixation on the target confirming a left convergent squint. **C.** The cover is removed and the left eye becomes convergent again.

(Fig. 118) in order to identify whether the squint is concomitant or incomitant. In concomitant squints, the deviation does not vary with different positions of gaze, whereas in incomitant squints the deviation does increase or decrease depending on which direction the eyes are looking. Incomitant squints are usually caused by disease of the muscles or nerve supply to the muscles and the affected eye demonstrates a reduction in movement in one or more direction.

Field of vision

A gross assessment of a patient's visual fields can be obtained by testing them clinically 'to confrontation', i.e. sitting opposite the patient and comparing your own field of vision to that of the patient. Test each eye in turn and ask the patient to cover the eye that is not being tested.

1. To test their right eye, they look directly into the doctor's left eye with their right eye to ensure that their fixation does not wander

2. The doctor's arm is outstretched to the side
3. Each field in four quadrants is tested by moving fingers in the superior and inferior areas of their nasal and temporal fields and asking the patient when they detect any movement or to count the number of fingers presented.

This form of visual field testing is most useful for picking up reasonably large 'neurological' field defects; more subtle defects (e.g. glaucoma) need more sophisticated computerised field analysis.

15.3 Ophthalmoscopy

It is important to be able to examine the retina in order to detect any retinal or optic disc pathology. This involves the use of the ophthalmoscope, which should be used systematically.

1. The patient is asked to look straight ahead (not at the ceiling) at a small object of interest and the patient's right eye is examined with your right eye and their left eye with your left eye.
2. Turn the ophthalmoscope on, set the lens to zero and stand back from the patient, looking through the peephole at the eye to observe the red reflex through the pupil.
3. Turn the lens to +10 (the plus lenses are usually the black numbers) and move in very close to the patient. This is now focused on the front of the eye (the anterior segment) and by working backwards through the lenses (+9, +8, +7, etc.), by turning the lens rack knob, the focus moves progressively further forward through the lens and vitreous humour onto the retina. By doing this it is possible to pick up opacities in the media, such as a cataract or a vitreous haemorrhage. It also means that a refractive error in either the patient or the examiner does not impair a good view of the retina, as one continues to turn the lens knob until a view of the fundus is obtained.
4. Examine the retina, looking first at the disc, then moving to the retinal vessels and periphery; examine the macular area last by asking the patient to look directly at the light.

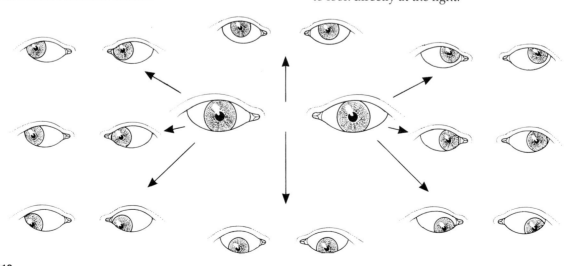

Fig. 118
The nine positions of gaze.

The eyelids and lacrimal system

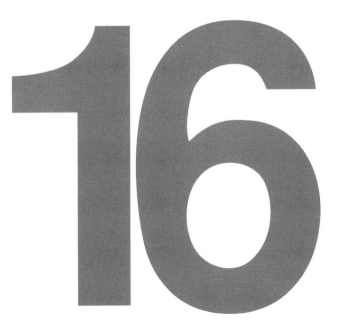

16.1 Introduction

The eyelids protect the eye and by their blinking action ensure that the tears are distributed evenly over the cornea.

Common lid problems are:

- eyelid infections
- abnormalities of eyelid position
- basal cell carcinoma.

Conditions of the lacrimal system discussed here are:

- kerato-conjunctivitis sicca (dry eyes)
- lacrimal outflow obstruction (watery eyes)
- dacryocystitis.

16.2 Eyelid infections

The eyelashes and eyelid meibomian glands are common sites of staphylococcal infection.

Hordeolum (stye)

This common cause of an acute inflammatory swelling of the eyelid is usually caused by staphylococcal infection of a lash follicle.

Clinical features
There is an acute red, tender swelling on the lid margin which 'points' along the lash line.

Management
Topical broad-spectrum antibiotics and steam bathing are used during the acute infection. Styes usually discharge spontaneously and resolve.

Chalazion

This swelling of the lid is caused by inflammation of the meibomian gland secondary to blockage of the gland duct.

Clinical features
A localised swelling occurs on the lid, just above the lash line; this may be inflamed, red and painful in the acute phase but may present as a painless solitary subcutaneous swelling.

Management
An acute chalazion often discharges spontaneously. Secondary infection should be treated with topical antibiotics. Incision and curettage is the definitive treatment of chronic chalazia.

Complications

- secondary infection

- incomplete resolution resulting in a chronic focus of granulomatous inflammation that may persist as a painless swelling for many months.

Chronic blepharitis

Blepharitis is a chronic inflammation of the lid margins and is a common cause of chronic ocular irritation. It may develop spontaneously for no known reason or be associated with acne rosacea, eczema or psoriasis.

Clinical features
The lid margins are red and there may be crusting around the lashes in severe disease. This is a chronic disease in which the eyes are persistently gritty and sore.

Management
The lids should be cleaned using cotton buds dipped in a dilute solution of sodium bicarbonate or baby shampoo to remove the crusts and topical antibiotic ointment should be rubbed into the lid margins. If local measures are ineffective, and in those with acne rosacea, systemic tetracycline is recommended. Artificial tear supplements may be required. Any secondary infection or associated skin condition should be treated appropriately.

Complications
Patients are more likely to develop chalazia, an abnormal tear film, secondary conjunctivitis and keratitis.

16.3 Lid abnormalities

Ptosis

Drooping of the upper eyelid is known as ptosis and may be congenital or acquired. Causes include

- neurogenic causes
  — third cranial nerve palsy
  — Horner's syndrome (see Fig. 155)
- myogenic causes
  — weakness of the levator muscle (commonest cause of 'senile ptosis')
  — myasthenia gravis
- mechanical causes
  — cysts or swelling of the upper lid.

Clinical features
The upper lid usually overlies the cornea by 1 mm; in ptosis, this position is lower than normal. The diagnosis is made clinically by measuring the interpalpebral distance in each eye, i.e. the distance between the upper and lower lids.

Management
Any underlying cause should be managed appropri-

ately. In congenital ptosis, surgical correction is required only if the visual axis is occluded, otherwise surgery is deferred until the child is due to go to school. As ptosis may induce astigmatism, all affected children should be referred to an ophthalmologist. Surgery usually consists of attaching the upper lid to the brow using a subcutaneous sling.

Surgery in acquired ptosis is carried out for cosmetic reasons and consists of shortening the levator muscle.

Complications

In affected children, the eye is at risk of developing 'deprivation amblyopia' if the eyelid droops enough to cover the visual axis (the centre of the pupil). Deprivation amblyopia is a condition in which the vision in one or both eyes does not develop properly because they are deprived of normal visual stimuli. This may be the result of a variety of causes, such as a droopy lid or a congenital cataract occluding the visual axis.

Lower lid entropion

In entropion, the eyelid turns in and the lashes abrade the cornea. The most common cause is senile laxity of the lower lid tissues. Congenital cases (epiblepheron) are usually self-limiting.

Clinical features

This is usually a condition of the elderly. The lashes rub on the cornea and conjunctiva causing redness, pain and the feeling that there is something in the eye. If it is not obvious, it may be necessary to ask the patient to forcibly close the eye and then open it to induce the entropion.

Management

Surgical correction to evert the lid to its normal position.

Complications

- bacterial conjunctivitis
- corneal abrasion.

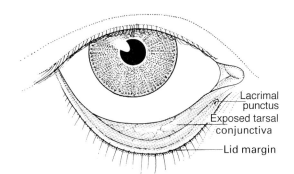

Fig. 119
Lower lid ectropion.

Lower lid ectropion

In ectropion (Fig. 119), the lower lid turns out and the exposed tarsal conjunctiva becomes inflamed. This is usually a result of senile laxity of the orbicularis muscle and the other lid tissues.

Clinical features

The eye is uncomfortable because of exposure of the lower aspect of the cornea. The eye may water because the lower lacrimal punctum is everted.

Management

Treatment is surgical and is aimed at reducing the laxity of the lid.

Complications

- bacterial conjunctivitis
- exposure keratitis.

16.4 Lid tumours

Basal cell carcinoma

As the eyelid skin is exposed to sunlight, basal cell carcinoma (BCC) is the most commonly seen tumour, representing 95% of eyelid malignancies. Other eyelid tumours include squamous cell carcinoma and malignant melanoma.

Clinical features

BCCs are usually raised lesions with a pearly margin and an ulcerated centre. The most common sites around the eye are the lower lid and medial canthal region. The clinical diagnosis is confirmed by biopsy.

Management

Management is by surgical excision, cryotherapy, or radiotherapy.

Both methods have similar success rates; however, local excision is usually preferred since complete surgical clearance can be confirmed histologically.

Complications

The tumour is locally invasive and can penetrate deep into the orbit, but it does not metastasise.

16.5 Lacrimal system

Lacrimal outflow obstruction (watery eyes)

Tears drain from the conjunctival sac through the lacrimal puncta and canaliculi into the lacrimal sac in the medial wall of the orbit. From there they drain down the nasolacrimal duct to its opening in the nose beneath the inferior turbinate (Fig. 120). Obstruction at any point along this pathway results in epiphora (watering of the eye). This may be congenital or acquired.

Congenital nasolacrimal duct obstruction

Incomplete canalisation of the nasolacrimal duct leaves a membranous obstruction at its distal end. There is, therefore, no communication between the duct and the nose.

Clinical features

The eye waters from birth (congenital epiphora) and may be intermittently sticky but is rarely red or inflamed. In the vast majority of children (>90%), the membranous obstruction opens spontaneously during the first year of life and the symptoms resolve quickly and completely.

Management

The affected infant's mother is reassured that this is a self-limiting condition and is advised to clean the eye regularly and to massage the lacrimal sac to express any stagnant contents. Since there is a such a high rate of spontaneous resolution, surgery is only considered if epiphora persists beyond 1 year of age. Surgery consists of a probe being passed down the nasolacrimal duct to open the obstruction.

Complications

Occasionally there may be a secondary conjunctivitis.

Acquired lacrimal outflow obstruction

The cause of acquired obstruction of the lacrimal outflow system may be:

- idiopathic (in the majority of cases)
- infection (bacterial, viral, fungal)
- inflammation
- trauma.

Clinical features

There is painless watering of the eye, which may be worse in cold winds.

Management

Treatment is surgical. The obstruction is bypassed by creating a direct communication between the lacrimal sac and the nasal mucosa (dacryocystorhinostomy).

Complications

The most common complication is secondary infection: conjunctivitis, acute or chronic dacryocystitis (lacrimal sac infection).

Keratoconjunctivitis sicca (dry eyes)

The tears lubricate the ocular surface and contain antibacterial substances that protect against infection.

Keratoconjunctivitis sicca is an extremely common cause of ocular discomfort, especially in the elderly.

The underlying pathology is atrophy and fibrosis of the lacrimal gland caused by:

- senile changes in the lacrimal gland
- connective tissue diseases, e.g. Sjögren's syndrome, which is characterised by keratoconjunctivitis sicca, dry mouth and an autoimmune disease such as rheumatoid arthritis.

Clinical features

The patient complains that the eyes feel very dry and gritty. Paradoxically, the eyes may water from reflex secretion because of the irritation.

Schirmer's test demonstrates reduced tear production by placing small strips of filter paper into the lower fornix. However, this test can be unreliable and a better test is to examine the height of the tear strip at the lid margin (Fig. 121). Multiple small epithelial defects of the corneal and conjunctival epithelium are evident on slit lamp examination.

Management

Artificial tear-drops and lubricating ointments provide symptomatic relief. Secondary infection is treated with antibiotics.

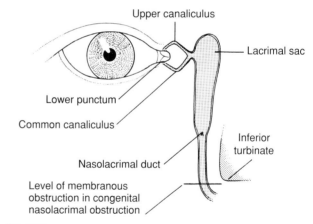

Fig. 120
The lacrimal drainage system.

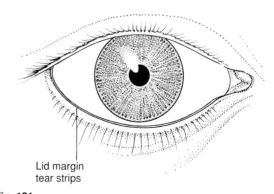

Fig. 121
Marginal tear strips can be seen at the lid margins. A drop of fluorescein makes these tear strips bright yellow when illuminated using a blue light.

Complications

- bacterial conjunctivitis or keratitis
- reduced vision because of the corneal epithelial changes.

Dacryocystitis

Dacryocystitis is an infection of the lacrimal sac, often secondary to acquired nasolacrimal duct obstruction, which may be acute or chronic.

Clinical features

Acute dacryocystitis. This is an extremely painful, tender, red swelling at the medial canthus. Pus builds up in the lacrimal sac and without treatment discharges through the skin.

Chronic dacryocystitis. Chronic infection causes a painless swelling of the sac. Mucopurulent material accumulates in the sac and can be expressed through the lacrimal puncta by pressure on the swelling.

Management

Acute dacryocystitis requires systemic antibiotics, whereas chronic dacryocystitis requires surgery (dacryocystorhinostomy).

Self-assessment: questions

Multiple choice questions

1. Lower lid entropion:
   a. Is associated with facial nerve paralysis
   b. Is treated surgically
   c. Is common in the elderly
   d. May be treated by removing the lashes
   e. Is a cause of corneal abrasion

2. Congenital epiphora
   a. Is caused by infection
   b. Has a high spontaneous resolution rate
   c. Should be treated urgently by probing the nasolacrimal duct
   d. May be associated with conjunctivitis
   e. Is associated with amblyopia

Case history

A 65-year-old female has had a watery eye for some years. Over the last 3 days, she has developed a painful tender swelling at the medial aspect of the orbit. The swelling is red and was very tender to touch until there was a discharge of green pus though the skin this morning.

1. What is the likely diagnosis?
2. What is the treatment?

Short notes

Write short notes on the following:

1. basal cell carcinoma
2. acute hordeolum
3. dry eyes

Self-assessment: answers

Multiple choice answers

1. a. **False.** Facial nerve paralysis is a cause of ectropion, not entropion, as it causes laxity of the orbicularis oculi muscle.
   b. **True.** Surgery everts the lid to its normal position.
   c. **True.** As a result of senile laxity of the lower lid tissues.
   d. **False.** If the lashes are removed they grow again and the small growing lashes abrade the cornea more.
   e. **True.**

2. a. **False.** It results from incomplete canalisation of the nasolacrimal duct.
   b. **True.**
   c. **False.** Because of the high spontaneous resolution, probing is not indicated in the first year.
   d. **True.** Secondary conjunctivitis is a possible complication.
   e. **False.** There is no known association with amblyopia.

Case history answer

1. The diagnosis is acute dacryocystitis.
2. Treatment is with systemic antibiotics and once the infection has resolved a dacryocystorhinostomy may be required if the eye continues to water or if chronic infection occurs.

Short notes answers

1. Basal cell carcinoma is the most common eyelid tumour. The most important aetiological factor is exposure to sunlight. Basal cell carcinoma commonly arises on the lower lid or medial canthal region. The tumour is usually raised with a pearly margin and an ulcerated centre. The tumour is locally invasive and must be completely removed. Treatment is with radiotherapy or surgical excision.
2. An acute hordeolum is an acute staphylococcal infection of one of the eyelash follicles. It causes an acute, red swelling of the lid that is tender and may discharge at the lid margin. Treatment is with topical antibiotics.
3. Keratoconjunctivitis sicca (dry eyes) is a very common problem, especially in the elderly. It is caused by reduced tear production because of atrophy of the lacrimal gland. The most common causes are ageing, atrophy of the lacrimal gland and Sjögren's syndrome, which comprises dry eyes, dry mouth and an autoimmune disorder, of which rheumatoid arthritis is the commonest. The eyes feel dry and gritty. Dry eyes may be complicated by bacterial conjunctivitis, corneal abrasion and bacterial keratitis. Treatment is with artificial tear-drops and lubricating ointments.

The conjunctiva, cornea and sclera

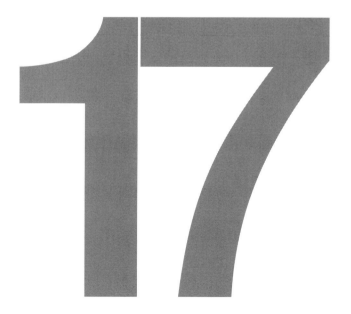

17.1 The conjunctiva

The conjunctiva is a mucous membrane covering the inner surface of the eyelids and the globe (excluding the cornea). The most common diseases of the conjunctiva are infective and allergic conjunctivitis.

Infection

Acute conjunctivitis caused by bacterial, viral or chlamydial infection is a bilateral condition that is characterised by ocular redness, discomfort and discharge.

Bacterial conjunctivitis

Bacterial infection causes a purulent conjunctivitis. The most common pathogens are staphylococci, streptococci and *Haemophilus influenzae*.

Clinical features
The patient gives a history of an acute onset of red, gritty eyes with a purulent discharge that characteristically causes the eyelids to be stuck together on wakening. The redness is diffuse and maximal deep in the conjunctival fornices rather than around the cornea. The vision is normal.

Diagnosis
The diagnosis is usually made on clinical grounds, although pathogenic organisms may be identified by culture of conjunctival swabs.

Management
Treatment is with a broad-spectrum topical antibiotic drop or ointment, such as chloramphenicol.

Adenovirus conjunctivitis

Adenovirus is a common cause of acute conjunctivitis with keratitis (inflammation of the cornea). Other viral causes of conjunctivitis include herpes simplex and molluscum contagiosum.

Clinical features
Although bilateral, this infection is commonly asymmetrical. The eyes are red with a watery discharge and mild photophobia. The preauricular lymph node is often enlarged and tender.

Diagnosis
The diagnosis is based on clinical findings. Viral swabs may be used to confirm the diagnosis.

Management
Antiviral agents are ineffective and treatment is mainly supportive. Antibiotics are usually prescribed to reduce the risk of secondary infection. The condition is highly contagious and the patient should be advised on strict hygiene, e.g. not sharing a face towel with another family member.

Complications

- keratitis
- secondary bacterial conjunctivitis.

The associated keratitis takes the form of punctate lesions over the entire cornea, which resolve slowly over some months. They are not usually associated with reduced vision.

Chlamydial conjunctivitis

Conjunctivitis caused by *Chlamydia trachomatis* can be divided into two distinct groups, trachoma and sexually transmitted conjunctivitis.

- Trachoma — this infection is common in the Third World as it occurs in areas of poor sanitation. It affects approximately four million people worldwide and is one of the leading causes of preventable blindness
- Sexually transmitted conjunctivitis — this condition tends to affect young adults. An acute or chronic, bilateral conjunctivitis develops approximately 2 weeks after sexual exposure. The eyes are red, the discharge is purulent and there is slight, non-tender enlargement of the preauricular lymph nodes. This is usually not sight-threatening.

Diagnosis
The diagnosis can be confirmed by detecting antibodies to chlamydia in the tears or serum. Alternatively, cytoplasmic inclusion bodies may be detected in scrapings of the conjunctival epithelium.

Management
Treatment is with systemic and topical tetracycline or erythromycin. As the infection is sexually transmitted, all patients must be referred to a genitourinary physician. Contact tracing is required to ensure treatment of sexual partners; failure to do so may result in reinfection or further spread of the infection.

Complications

- keratitis is very common
- chronic conjunctival and corneal scarring occurs if the infection is inadequately treated or the patient becomes recurrently reinfected.

Neonatal conjunctivitis (ophthalmia neonatorum)

This is an acute conjunctivitis occurring in the first month of life. It is a notifiable disease. The usual source of infection is the mother's genital tract and the most common causative organisms are staphylococci and chlamydia. Gonococcal infections are very rare but may cause severe conjunctivitis.

Clinical features
The child develops an acute purulent conjunctivitis, the lids may be swollen and the eyes closed.

Diagnosis
Bacteriological investigations are mandatory. Conjunctival swabs are cultured for bacterial organisms, including gonococci and for chlamydia.

Management
Bacterial infections resolve quickly with topical antibiotics. In chlamydial infection, systemic antibiotics, e.g. erythromycin, are required. The mother requires treatment and contact tracing for any genital tract infection.

Complications
- chlamydial neonatal conjunctivitis is often associated with a pneumonitis.
- gonococcal infection may lead to corneal perforation.

Allergic conjunctivitis

The hallmark of allergy is itch. The most common important manifestations are hay fever conjunctivitis and vernal conjunctivitis.

Hay fever conjunctivitis

Hay fever conjunctivitis is a very common self-limiting acute conjunctivitis associated with type 1 immediate hypersensitivity to pollens.

Clinical features
The eyes become acutely red and itchy. There is marked oedema and swelling of the conjunctiva. The condition is often seasonal and patients are usually atopic (a history of asthma and eczema).

Diagnosis
The diagnosis is clinical. Patch testing may be useful in identifying a particular antigen.

Management
Topical antihistamines may be of benefit during the acute reaction.

Vernal keratoconjunctivitis (spring catarrh)

Vernal keratoconjunctivitis is an allergic condition of children and young adults and is caused by the release of inflammatory mediators from conjunctival mast cells and basophils, causing bilateral ocular inflammation.

Clinical features
The outstanding symptom is intense ocular itch. The eyes water and there is a tenacious mucous discharge. Exacerbations occur in the Spring. Boys are more commonly affected than girls. There is a tendency to spontaneous remission in adolescence, but this is not always the case. There is an association with atopy.

Management
Treatment is with mast cell stabilisers such as sodium cromoglycate drops. Steroids are only used during acute exacerbations. Steroids should not be used in the long term as they are associated with a risk of glaucoma, cataract and potentiation of infection; if indicated, they must only be used under ophthalmic supervision.

Complications
Keratitis is the most serious and potentially sight-threatening complication.

17.2 The cornea

The cornea (see Fig. 115) is the major refracting structure of the eye and its clarity is essential for good vision. The corneal stroma is continuous with the white sclera, which is covered by the highly vascular episcleral tissue. The corneal epithelium is continuous with the conjunctiva. The major disorders affecting the cornea are keratitis and keratoconus. The episcleral tissue may become inflamed, causing episcleritis. Scleritis, or inflammation of the sclera, is an uncommon but serious condition.

Keratitis and corneal ulceration

Keratitis is any inflammatory or infective process affecting the cornea. When the epithelial surface is deficient, which is usually localised, this is termed a corneal ulcer.

Marginal keratitis

This is the most common inflammatory condition affecting the cornea. It is caused by hypersensitivity to staphylococcal exotoxins and is often seen in patients with blepharitis.

Clinical features
The patient complains of a painful eye with photophobia. There is an epithelial defect adjacent to the limbus, called a marginal ulcer, which stains with fluorescein. The adjacent conjunctiva and episclera are hyperaemic.

Management
The condition is usually self-limiting but resolves more quickly with a mild topical steroid.

Bacterial keratitis

Although primary infection may occur, the corneal epithelium is generally a good barrier to infection. Therefore, infection is usually associated with a predisposing factor, such as:

- trauma (corneal abrasion)

- contact lens wear
- corneal anaesthesia resulting from neurological disease
- keratoconjunctivitis sicca.

The most common bacterial pathogens are staphylococci and the Gram-negative organisms.

Clinical features

The condition is usually unilateral. The patient presents with an acute red eye associated with watering or a purulent discharge. There is intense pain and photophobia, the vision is reduced particularly if the ulcer is in the centre of the cornea. The corneal epithelial defect may be easily visualised under blue light following instillation of fluorescein drops. There is a secondary anterior uveitis, and inflammatory pus cells may settle in the inferior aspect of the anterior chamber, causing a white fluid level known as a 'hypopyon'.

Diagnosis

The causative organism is identified by microscopy and culture of conjunctival swabs and scrapings from the corneal ulcer.

Management

The patient may require hospital admission for urgent and intensive treatment with topical or subconjunctival antibiotics to treat the infection. This should limit scarring and prevent the catastrophic complication of corneal perforation.

Complications

- anterior uveitis
- permanent reduction in vision from scarring
- corneal perforation may occur.

Herpes simplex (dendritic ulcer)

Exposure to herpes simplex virus is very common, with 90% of the adult population showing antibodies to the virus. The virus remains latent in the trigeminal ganglion and may become reactivated, causing a dendritic ulcer.

Clinical features

The hallmark of herpes simplex keratitis is dendritic ulceration of the corneal epithelium (Fig. 122). The eye is painful and red, with watering, photophobia and reduced vision.

Diagnosis

Herpes simplex can be cultured from viral swabs, but commonly the diagnosis is made on the clinical features of a dendritic ulcer that stains with fluorescein.

Management

Treatment is with antiviral ointment, e.g. acyclovir. Topical steroids must not be prescribed; they dampen the inflammatory response, making the eye more comfortable, but the ulcer becomes larger and deeper resulting in severe scarring and permanent reduction in vision. Because of this risk, patients with an acute red eye should not be given topical steroids except under the supervision of an ophthalmologist.

Complications

The condition is frequently recurrent and may lead to corneal scarring. As the virus inhabits the nerve, reduction in corneal sensation is almost universal following recurrent attacks of herpes simplex keratitis.

Keratoconus

In this condition, the cornea develops a conical contour or shape. The cause is unknown; however, keratoconus is more common in atopic individuals and those with Down's syndrome and may result from constant rubbing of the eyes.

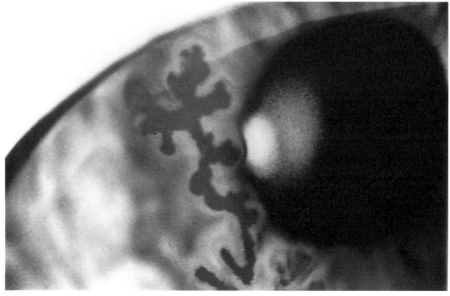

Fig. 122
Dendritic ulcer.

Clinical features

The patients usually present around puberty or early adult life because of blurring of vision in one or both eyes. This is caused by the development of irregular astigmatism, which increases as the cornea becomes more conical.

Management

Initially the visual acuity may be improved with spectacles, but usually contact lenses are required to correct the high degree of astigmatism. Corneal grafting may be required later if contact lenses can no longer be fitted or the cornea becomes scarred.

Complications

Sudden onset of a localised area of corneal oedema or scarring at the tip of the cone, which cause marked reduction in vision.

17.3 The sclera

Episcleritis

This is a is a self-limiting inflammation of the episcleral tissue of unknown aetiology. The condition is more common in females.

Clinical features

The patient complains of mild irritation, usually in one eye. The affected eye usually appears red in the inter-palpebral area (Fig. 123). Two forms exist: nodular and diffuse episcleritis. In the nodular type, there is a raised yellow nodule on the episclera with surrounding hyperaemia. In the diffuse type, there is no nodule but diffuse hyperaemia occurs.

Management

The condition usually resolves spontaneously within 10 to 14 days. Resolution may be hastened by a mild topical steroid under ophthalmic supervision.

Scleritis

This is a rare inflammation of the sclera that tends to affect older patients, usually females. Causes may be:

- idiopathic
- connective tissue diseases, of which rheumatoid arthritis is the most common.

Clinical features

The most characteristic feature is severe ocular pain, which serves to differentiate scleritis from episcleritis. The sclera becomes intensely red, either diffusely or in one quadrant.

Management

The mainstay of treatment is topical and systemic steroids.

Complications

Scleritis is a serious type of ocular inflammation that may result in permanent reduction in vision. The underlying aetiology is a vasculitis affecting the scleral vessels. The sclera becomes inflamed and thin. 'Scleromalacia perforans' is a condition in which the eye perforates in an area of necrotic sclera (usually in patients with rheumatoid arthritis).

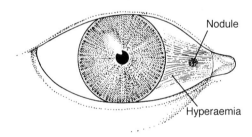

Fig. 123
Episcleritis affecting the nasal interpalpebral zone.

Self-assessment: questions

Multiple choice questions

1. Vernal conjunctivitis:
   a. Is rarely sight-threatening
   b. Is characterised by a purulent discharge
   c. Is more common in males
   d. Is characterised by intense ocular itch
   e. Is treated for prolonged periods with topical steroids

2. Chlamydial conjunctivitis:
   a. Rarely causes keratitis
   b. May cause neonatal conjunctivitis
   c. In neonates is associated with pneumonitis
   d. Is treated with topical antibiotics
   e. Is sexually transmitted

3. Herpes simplex keratitis:
   a. Is usually treated with topical steroids in the acute phase
   b. Is associated with a purulent discharge
   c. Is characterised by a dendritic corneal ulcer
   d. Is a recurrent disease
   e. Is more common in contact lens wearers

Case histories

History 1

A young mother brings a 14-day-old girl to the clinic with a sticky red eye. The eyelids are swollen and closed.

1. What is the diagnosis?
2. What organisms may cause this infection?
3. How is the diagnosis confirmed?
4. How would the problem be managed?

History 2

A 30-year-old management executive has had an acute red eye for 4 days. The patient normally wears soft contact lenses and thinks he may have hurt the eye putting the lenses in. The eyes are stuck together in the mornings because of a green discharge, and for the last 24 hours the pain has become severe and vision reduced. On examination, the eye is extremely red and there is a central corneal epithelial defect. There is a white opacity under the epithelial defect and a hypopyon.

1. What is the likely diagnosis?
2. What factors predispose to infection?
3. How should this patient be managed?
4. What complications may occur?

Short notes

Write short notes on the following:

1. viral conjunctivitis
2. chlamydial conjunctivitis
3. keratoconus
4. episcleritis

Self-assessment: answers

Multiple choice answers

1. a. **False.** Vernal conjunctivitis may be complicated by keratitis, which is sight-threatening.
   b. **False.** Purulent discharge is associated with infection, not allergy.
   c. **True.**
   d. **True.** This is the outstanding symptom.
   e. **False.** Topical steroids must only be used for short periods of time because of the risk of glaucoma, cataract and infection.

2. a. **False.** Keratitis is a common feature of chlamydial infection.
   b. **True.** Because the condition is sexually transmitted, an affected mother may pass the infection to her offspring during childbirth from her infected genital tract.
   c. **True.**
   d. **False.** Chlamydial infection is systemic and, therefore, requires systemic antibiotics.
   e. **True.** Contact tracing is required to ensure treatment of sexual partners to prevent reinfection or the further spread of infection.

3. a. **False.** Topical steroids potentiate infection and are absolutely contraindicated in the acute phase.
   b. **False.** Herpes simplex keratitis is associated with a watery discharge.
   c. **True.**
   d. **True.** Herpes simplex remains latent in the trigeminal ganglion and may become reactivated.
   e. **False.** Recurrence is not related to contact lens wear.

Case history answers

History 1

1. The clinical diagnosis is neonatal conjunctivitis, since the child is only 14 days old.
2. The infection is commonly caused by bacteria or chlamydia.
3. Conjunctival swabs are taken for culture and detection of antibodies to chlamydia.
4. Intensive broad-spectrum antibiotics are started initially. If chlamydia is later confirmed, systemic treatment is required with erythromycin and the child should be seen by a paediatrician because of the risk of pneumonitis. In chlamydial conjunctivitis, the source of infection is the mother's genital tract. She must be referred to the genitourinary clinic for investigation and contact tracing.

History 2

1. The likely diagnosis is bacterial keratitis because there is a purulent discharge, an epithelial defect and a hypopyon.
2. The major predisposing factor is soft contact lens wear. The patient may not take care of the lenses and admits that he has difficulty putting the lens into the eye.
3. The patient should be admitted for intensive antibiotic drops. Conjunctival swabs should be cultured and scrapings of the ulcer examined and cultured for organisms.
4. There is usually an anterior uveitis. Rarely, corneal perforation may occur.

Short notes answers

1. Adenovirus causes an acute conjunctivitis. The eyes are red with watering and photophobia. The infection may be preceded by upper respiratory tract infection and fever, especially in children. Complications include keratitis and secondary bacterial conjunctivitis. The keratitis takes the form of punctate lesions over the entire cornea, which slowly resolve. Treatment is supportive and topical antibiotics are given to stop secondary bacterial infection.
2. This is a sexually transmitted disease mainly affecting young adults. It may also cause neonatal conjunctivitis. There is an acute or chronic bilateral purulent conjunctivitis 2 weeks after sexual exposure. Complications include keratitis and, in neonates, pneumonitis. Treatment is with systemic antibiotics: tetracycline in adults and erythromycin in neonates. Contact tracing is mandatory.
3. In keratoconus the cornea has a conical shape. Although the cause is unknown, it is more common in atopic patients and patients with Down's syndrome. The patient presents in early adult life with blurring of vision that gradually increases. Reduced vision is caused by astigmatism and may be corrected initially with spectacles and then by contact lenses. Eventually a corneal graft may be necessary, especially if the cornea has become scarred.
4. Episcleritis is a self-limiting condition that is more common in females and is of unknown aetiology. There is ocular discomfort and mild irritation. Two forms exist: nodular and diffuse episcleritis. In the nodular type, there is a raised yellow nodule on the episclera and a surrounding hyperaemia. The condition is self-limiting, usually resolving within 14 days. Resolution may be hastened by a mild topical steroid.

Refraction and the lens

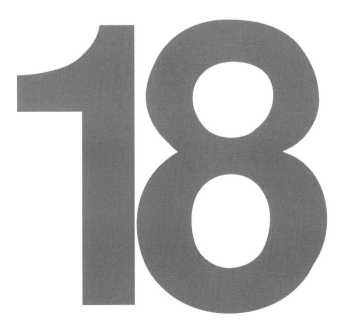

18.1 Physiology

Normally light from an object enters the eye and is focused on the fovea of the retina. The image of a distant object is brought to focus on the fovea through refraction by the cornea and lens (Fig. 124A). In order to see near objects clearly, a focusing mechanism is required (accommodation). On accommodation, the power of the lens is increased by contraction of the ciliary muscle (Fig. 120B). The majority of people have no refractive error, that is they have clear vision without the need of glasses. They are emmetropic. In refractive disorders, this is not the case and images are focused behind or in front of the retina. This results in blurred vision and the patient needs glasses in order to see clearly.

Common disorders of refraction are:

- myopia
- hypermetropia
- astigmatism
- presbyopia.

The lens is a biconvex structure situated behind the iris. It consists of a central nucleus surrounded by a peripheral cortex contained within a transparent membrane, the lens capsule. The lens is held in place by the lens zonules.

Disorders affecting the lens include:

- cataract, which may be acquired or congenital
- ectopia lentis (dislocation of the lens), which may be associated with a number of systemic conditions.

18.2 Disorders of refraction

Myopia (short sight)

In myopia, the eye is relatively longer than normal and the image of a distant object is brought to focus in front of the retina. Distance vision is reduced but can be corrected by using a concave (diverging) spectacle lens. These people have good near vision, hence the term short sight (Fig. 125).

Hypermetropia (long sight)

In hypermetropia, the eye is relatively shorter than normal and the image of a distant object is behind the retina. A convex (converging) spectacle will correct this. If the degree of hypermetropia is not great, then this may be achieved by accommodation, so that most young people with mild hypermetropia have good distance vision, even without glasses (Fig. 126).

Astigmatism

The refractive power of the cornea is dependent upon its curvature. In astigmatism, the corneal curvature is

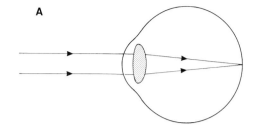

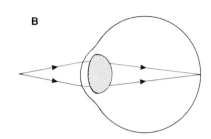

Fig. 124
A. Normal eye. Emmetropia. **B.** Accommodation. The lens becomes thicker to increase its power, which allows focus on a near object.

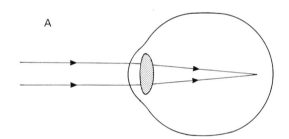

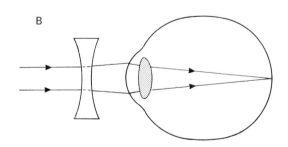

Fig. 125
A. Myopia. **B.** Corrective lens for myopia.

not uniform, making it impossible to bring an image into sharp focus on the retina. The usual description given to patients is that the surface of the eye is more like a rugby ball than the normal eye, which is more football shaped. The vision is blurred, but an astigmatic spectacle lens, which neutralises the differences in corneal curvature, will correct this (Fig. 127).

Irregular astigmatism is an uneven surface of the

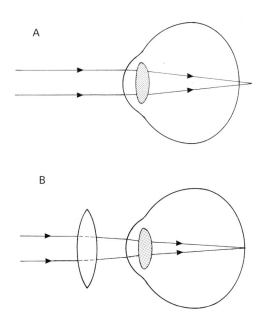

Fig. 126
A. Hypermetropia. **B.** Corrective lens for hypermetropia.

cornea resulting from corneal scarring or keratoconus and cannot be corrected by glasses.

Presbyopia

Accommodation for near work is dependent upon the plasticity of the lens. With increasing age, the lens becomes more rigid and it cannot change shape so easily. The ability to focus for close work, therefore, decreases with age so that books, papers, etc. have to be held progressively further away. This is a normal process termed 'presbyopia'. Reading glasses are required in order to focus on a near object, usually from about the age of 40 onwards.

Overcoming refractive errors

A simple method of determining whether reduced vision is caused by a refractive error is to demonstrate that the acuity improves with the use of a pin-hole. The patient looks through a tiny pin-hole made in a piece of card; if the eye is healthy other than a refractive error, the vision will improve. Formal testing for spectacles, or 'refraction', necessitates more complex assessment and is carried out by an optometrist or ophthalmologist.

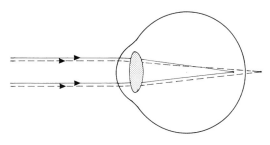

Fig. 127
Astigmatism. No point focus is formed.

Treatment of refractive disorders
There are a number of methods used to treat refractive errors:

- spectacle correction is the traditional method of improving vision
- contact lenses are preferred by some patients; rigid lenses (gas permeable) or soft lenses
- corneal refractive surgery is a new method of treating refactive errors; it is in its early stages and is still considered to be 'experimental' by some. This can be carried out using radial corneal incisions or laser treatment of the cornea. These treatments are irreversible and also expensive.

18.3 Disorders of the lens

Cataract

A cataract is an opacity in the lens. This is a very common cause of poor vision, especially in the older age groups. Cataract is commonly situated in one of three portions of the lens. An opacity in the central portion of the lens is termed nuclear sclerosis. Cataract in the periphery of the lens has a radial spoke-like pattern and is called cortical cataract. An opacity at the posterior aspect of the lens is called a posterior subcapsular cataract; this type of cataract can be particularly visually disabling.

Senile cataracts are the most common type, but secondary cataracts do develop as a result of:

- ocular trauma
- ocular disease, e.g. uveitis
- metabolic disorders: diabetes is the most common, galactosaemia and hypercalcaemia are rare
- drugs: notably prolonged use of systemic steroids
- congenital and hereditary cataract.

Clinical features
The patient presents with gradual, painless reduction in vision over a period of months to years. Occasionally the complaint is also of glare, especially under bright conditions. The cataract may be observed as a disturbance of the red reflex on ophthalmoscopy or, in severe disease, as a white pupil (leucocoria).

Management
The only effective way to deal with cataract is to surgically remove the opacified lens. There is no critical level of visual acuity considered appropriate for surgery. This should be performed once the vision is reduced to the point where the patient is experiencing problems because of poor vision.

Cataract extraction is the most common ocular operation performed today. Methods of cataract extraction are:

- intracapsular cataract extraction (ICCE)
- extracapsular cataract extraction (ECCE)

• phaco-emulsification (a modified type of ECCE).

Intracapsular extraction. The lens is removed intact, i.e. the lens capsule and its contents are extracted in entirety. Because the powerful lens has been removed, this causes profound blurring of vision that requires correction with very strong spectacle lenses. These are associated with many optical aberrations because of their thickness, which commonly results in spectacle intolerance. Contact lenses do not cause these optical problems but are inconvenient to use, particularly in the elderly. This technique is rarely employed in the UK today but is a rapid, inexpensive method and is used to remove cataracts in developing countries.

Extracapsular extraction. This involves removal of the lens nucleus and cortex from the capsule, leaving the capsule intact (except for a hole in the anterior surface that is used to remove the contents). This is less disrupting for the eye than ICCE. The major advantage of this technique is that the remaining capsule can be used to hold a replacement artificial, plastic intraocular lens, which is permanently implanted into the eye at the time of surgery (Figs 128 and 129). These lenses are available in different refractive powers, and the power of the implant is determined preoperatively to give the patient clear vision for distance. Spectacles are usually still required for reading or near work.

Phaco-emulsification. This is a newer method of extracapsular surgery using a 'key-hole' incision. The lens capsule is opened and the contents are broken up by a small oscillating 'phaco-tip' and removed piecemeal. A small or foldable intraocular lens is implanted through the 2–3 mm incision and no sutures are required to close the wound (Fig. 130). This technique allows rapid patient rehabilitation and has better visual results because of the small wound.

Postoperative care. Topical steroids and antibiotics are prescribed routinely after cataract surgery to prevent infection and reduce inflammation.

Complications of cataracts. Cataracts cause an uncomplicated reduction in vision, although if left too long, they become 'mature'. This means that the lens may swell up, causing intraocular inflammation and increased intraocular pressure.

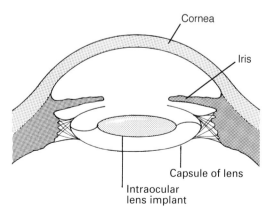

Fig. 128
Intraocular lens implant inside the lens capsule at the end of an operation.

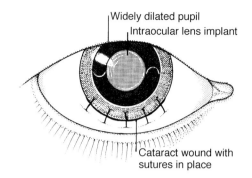

Fig. 129
View of an extracapsular operation at the end of surgery.

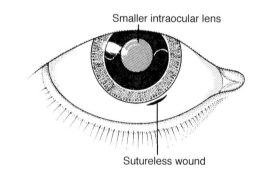

Fig. 130
The surgeon's view of phaco-emulsification at the end of surgery. Note the small wound and intraocular lens.

Complications of cataract surgery
Common complications

• astigmatism induced by a wound that is either too tight or too loose (this is reduced with phaco-emulsification)
• postoperative uveitis; this is usually mild
• opacification of the capsule which holds the intraocular lens, causing a blurring of vision; this can be easily treated using a laser to disrupt an area of the capsule, making a clear hole in its centre.

Rare complications

• intraocular infection (endophthalmitis), which is visually devastating. The infection is usually acquired at the time of surgery
• retinal detachment
• corneal decompensation.

Congenital cataract

Congenital cataracts are a rare but important cause of blindness in childhood. They can cause profound loss of vision. They may be unilateral or bilateral.
  Causes include:

• idiopathic (> 50% of patients)
• intrauterine rubella infection

- inborn errors of metabolism: galactosaemia is the most common
- chromosome abnormalities such as Down's syndrome.

Clinical features

All infants should be screened routinely for the presence of lens opacities. This can be done by looking at the red reflex with a direct ophthalmoscope. In patients with advanced disease, the diagnosis is made more easily as the pupil appears white (leucocoria).

Management

The treatment of paediatric cataract is surgical. Surgery must be performed urgently as maturation of the visual system is dependent on clear vision from an early age. There will be profound and permanent visual loss (amblyopia) if the eye is not treated early enough (usually within days to weeks of birth).

Ectopia lentis

Ectopia lentis or lens subluxation occurs when the lens becomes dislocated or subluxated because of damage to the lens zonules.

Causes include:

- trauma
- idiopathic
- severe myopia
- Marfan's syndrome and homocystinurea are uncommon causes due to abnormal structure of the lens zonules.

Clinical features

The patient may have no complaints, or they may be aware of a sudden reduction in vision if the lens dislocates fully out of the visual axis.

Management

No treatment is required if the patient is asymptomatic; otherwise the entire lens should be removed and the patient's vision corrected, preferably with a contact lens.

Complications

- anterior dislocation of the lens into the anterior chamber, predisposing to acute glaucoma
- posterior dislocation of the lens, causing uveitis.

Self-assessment: questions

Multiple choice questions

1. Cataracts:
   a. Are more common in diabetics
   b. May be treated by drugs
   c. Are a cause of ocular pain
   d. Cause sudden loss of vision
   e. That are drug induced are often caused by systemic steroids

2. Which of the following are complications of cataract surgery:
   a. Retinal detachment
   b. Retinal vein occlusion
   c. Infection
   d. Uveitis
   e. Astigmatism

3. Cataract surgery:
   a. Is a common operation
   b. Is only required when the patient is blind
   c. Has no complications
   d. Is often carried out using the intracapsular method in this country
   e. Is often carried out using local anaesthesia

4. Which of the following become common as patients become older?
   a. Hypermetropia
   b. Myopia
   c. Cataract
   d. Presbyopia
   e. Astigmatism

Case history

A 67-year-old man attends the clinic complaining of gradual reduction in vision affecting both eyes. He is generally well and has never worn glasses. There is no family history of any eye diseases. Visual acuity is 6/24 in each eye, uncorrected, and does not improve with a pinhole.

1. What is the most likely diagnosis?
2. Discuss other possible diagnoses (information from other sections is required to answer this question).

Short notes

Write short notes on:

1. ectopia lentis
2. congenital cataract

Viva questions

1. What is the medical term for 'short sight'?
2. What type of spectacle lens would correct this?
3. When do people usually become presbyopic?
4. What are the symptoms of presbyopia?
5. What type of lens is used to treat this?
6. What methods are currently available for treating refractive errors?

Self-assessment: answers

Multiple choice answers

1. a. **True.** Diabetics are at increased risk of developing premature cataract.
   b. **False.** Surgery is the only effective method.
   c. **False.** Cataract does not cause pain in the eye.
   d. **False.** Cataract causes a gradual loss of vision.
   e. **True.** Prolonged use of systemic steroids can induce cataracts

2. a. **True.** A rare complication.
   b. **False.** Cataract surgery does not cause retinal vein occlusion.
   c. **True.** A rare complication.
   d. **True.** This is usually mild.
   e. **True.** Astigmatism is induced by a wound that is too tight or too loose.

3. a. **True.** Cataract surgery is the commonest ocular operation performed in this country and also worldwide.
   b. **False.** Patients require surgery when they are having visual difficulties due to their cataract. The measurement of visual acuity is not important and surgery should be carried out before the patient is blind.
   c. **False.** All operations have a complication rate.
   d. **False.** It is carried out using the extracapsular or phaco-emulsification techniques in this country. The intracapsular method is used in the developing countries.
   e. **True.** It is most commonly carried out using local anaesthesia as most patients are elderly, and most are also carried out as day cases.

4. a. **False.**
   b. **False.**
   c. **True.** Cataract is a condition of an ageing population.
   d. **True.** Patients become presbyopic in their 40s and 50s.
   e. **False.**

Case history answer

1. The most common cause of gradual deterioration of vision in this age group is cataract.

2. Other possible causes for these symptoms in a gentleman of this age are dry, age-related macular degeneration, or chronic open-angle glaucoma, which has advanced to a late stage.

Short notes answers

1. Ectopia lentis refers to a dislocation of the lens in the eye. This may be caused by trauma or, less commonly, the underlying cause is unknown or it is associated with Marfan's syndrome or homocystinuria. The patient may be unaware of any visual problems, although they may present with a deterioration of vision associated with another eye condition that predisposes them to dislocation of the lens. If the lens dislocates out of the visual axis, this is associated with a sudden deterioration in vision. Management involves observation and removal of the lens if any complications arise.
2. Congenital cataract is an important cause of visual disability in children. All infants should be screened for lens opacities as it is vital to remove a congenital cataract promptly to prevent deprivation amblyopia. This is often associated with other anomalies but may be an isolated finding.

Viva answers

1. Short sight is known as myopia.
2. A concave, or minus, lens is used to treat myopia.
3. Presbyopia usually becomes symptomatic at around 40 years of age.
4. The symptoms of presbyopia are (a) blurring of near vision and (b) having to hold books and other reading material further and further away in order to see them clearly.
5. A convex or plus lens is used to correct this.
6. Methods to treat refractive errors include (a) spectacles, (b) contact lenses and (c) refractive surgery.

The uveal tract, vitreous humour and retina

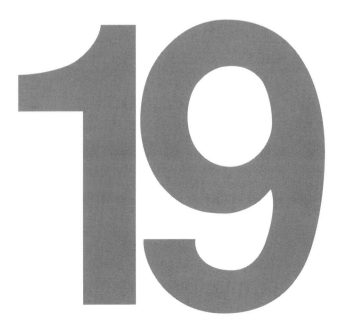

19.1 The uveal tract

The uveal tract is the middle layer of the eye, consisting of the iris, the ciliary body and the choroid. The iris is the anterior portion, which is a diaphragm that contains a central opening (the pupil) which controls the amount of light entering the eye. The ciliary body secretes aqueous humour and contains the ciliary muscle, which controls the focusing power of the lens. The choroid is the vascular layer of the posterior segment situated between the retina and the sclera.

The most important diseases involving the uveal tract are:

- uveitis
- malignant melanoma.

The retina is the innermost layer of the posterior segment of the eye. The most sensitive area of the retina is the fovea, situated at the centre of the macula at the posterior pole. The cones in this area are responsible for detailed vision, such as that involved in reading and colour perception. The peripheral retina is less sensitive to detail, but the rods in this part provide 'side vision' and good night vision. The vitreous humour is in the centre of the vitreous cavity. Abnormalities of these structures tend to affect the vision with no pain or redness.

Uveitis

Inflammatory conditions of the inner eye are referred to as 'uveitis'. These are usually divided into anterior uveitis (iritis) and posterior uveitis (choroiditis).

Acute anterior uveitis (iritis)

In more than 90% of patients, no underlying cause is found for the inflammation. Causes include:

- secondary to other eye diseases, such as corneal ulceration or retinal detachment
- following blunt trauma
- following cataract or glaucoma surgery
- in association with systemic inflammatory disorders, such as rheumatoid arthritis, ankylosing spondylitis, Reiter's disease, Crohn's disease, ulcerative colitis and sarcoidosis.

Clinical features

Acute iritis is usually unilateral and the patient presents with an extremely painful, red eye associated with photophobia and reduced vision.

Examination of the eye reveals ciliary (circumcorneal) injection; the pupil is usually small but may also be irregular because of adhesions between the anterior lens surface and the pupil margin (posterior synechia) (Fig. 131). Slit lamp examination is essential to make the diagnosis as this reveals increased protein (flare) and cells in the anterior chamber. A complete, detailed examination of the eye is required to reveal any underlying ocular cause for the condition.

Diagnosis

Investigations to identify the underlying cause are not usually carried out unless the condition becomes recurrent or there are clinical signs suggestive of an associated condition (e.g. low back pain or stiff joints).

Management

Management involves:

- topical steroid drops to reduce the inflammation
- cycloplegics (e.g. atropine drops) to relieve the intense pain which is caused by ciliary spasm and to prevent the development of posterior synechia.

Complications. Raised intraocular pressure may complicate acute iritis. Topical steroid treatment may also be complicated by a rise in intraocular pressure in susceptible individuals. The increased pressure may require treatment with antiglaucomatous medication (e.g. topical beta-blockers).

Chronic anterior uveitis (iritis)

Occasionally anterior uveitis lasts for several weeks and may persist for many years.

Causes include:

- idiopathic
- juvenile chronic arthritis, especially females with pauciarticular arthritis that is seronegative for rheumatoid factor but positive for antinuclear factor
- sarcoidosis.

Clinical features

In comparison with the acute form, chronic iritis often begins insidiously, and the patient may suffer few or no symptoms. Presenting features may consist of mild pain, blurring of vision or alternatively the presence of the disease may be picked up during routine eye examination. Children with juvenile arthritis must be examined regularly by an ophthalmologist to screen for any anterior segment inflammation.

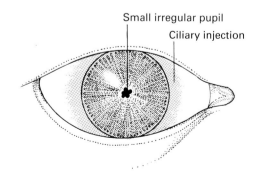

Small irregular pupil

Ciliary injection

Fig. 131
Anterior uveitis.

Chronic anterior uveitis may be a bilateral condition. The affected eyes are often white, but slit lamp examination reveals flare and cells in the anterior chamber, posterior synechia and microscopic condensations of cells on the posterior surface of the cornea (keratic precipitates).

Management

Management is with:

- steroid drops
- cycloplegic drops
- depot injections of steroid into the periocular tissues in severe disease
- systemic steroids in severe disease.

Complications. Long-term complications include loss of vision caused by:

- glaucoma
- macular oedema
- cataract
- corneal band keratopathy.

Posterior uveitis (choroiditis)

Causes of posterior uveitis include:

- congenital toxoplasmosis (which may reactivate at any time in adult life)
- other granulomatous infections, e.g. TB, syphilis
- toxocariasis
- autoimmune conditions, such as Behçet's or Wegener's disease, sarcoidosis
- idiopathic.

Clinical features

The patient complains of blurred vision, floaters and/or loss of vision, depending on the area of retinochoroidal damage. Posterior uveitis consists of vitreous cells and areas of focal retinal or choroidal damage. Such areas are seen as hazy, pale lesions on the posterior segment.

Diagnosis

Screening for active causative infections.

Management

This depends on the cause. Treatment is aimed at specific infective agents, and topical and systemic steroids are used to reduce the inflammatory response.

Tumours

The most common primary intraocular tumour is a malignant melanoma of the choroid. Secondaries from breast and lung tumours commonly metastasise to the choroid, but these frequently remain undiagnosed as they usually occur in the terminal stage of the disease.

Malignant melanoma

This tumour may occur in any age group but becomes more common with increasing age. These tumours often remain quiescent for long periods but may suddenly undergo a period of rapid growth. They arise from the melanocytes of the choroid.

Clinical features

The patient is commonly asymptomatic and the lesion is picked up at a screening ophthalmoscopy by an optician. On fundus examination, a raised pigmented or non-pigmented lesion is seen. There may be an associated retinal detachment, which gives rise to the symptoms of a field defect or reduced vision.

Diagnosis

Melanomas must be differentiated from benign naevi using an ultrasound examination of the posterior segment. Malignant melanomas have characteristic ultrasonic features. CT scanning is the best method of demonstrating extraocular extension.

Management

Management depends upon the size of the tumour and any documented growth.

Small tumours. Small tumours (especially in the elderly) should be observed for any signs of growth by regular clinical examination, photographs and ultrasound measurements.

Large tumours or those with evidence of growth. These may be treated with local cryotherapy, laser, radioactive plaques, external beam radiation, local surgical resection or enucleation (removal of the eye).

Large tumours with secondary retinal detachments. These require enucleation and those with evidence of extraocular spread should be exenterated (removal of the entire contents of the orbit).

Complications. Metastatic disease, especially to the liver.

19.2 The vitreous humour

Posterior vitreous detachment

The vitreous humour is attached to the retina in young people. With increasing age, the vitreous humour degenerates by liquefaction, becomes less formed and detaches from the retina. This tends to occur prematurely in myopic or traumatised eyes.

Clinical features

The patient complains of a transparent 'floater' in their field of vision.

The retinal periphery should be examined in detail to exclude retinal holes. If no pathology is found, the patient should be reassured as this is a normal physiological condition.

Complications

- as the vitreous humour detaches it may pull a small area of retina with it creating a retinal hole which predisposes to a retinal detachment
- vitreous haemorrhage.

Vitreous haemorrhage

Causes of vitreous haemorrhage include:

- posterior vitreous detachment
- retinal detachment
- retinal neovascularisation (secondary to retinal vein occlusion or diabetes)
- trauma.

Clinical features

Patients present with the sudden onset of dark floaters, which may become confluent. The vision is commonly reduced. Ophthalmoscopy reveals a reduced or absent red reflex with poor or no fundal details.

Management

Initially, time should be allowed for the haemorrhage to resolve spontaneously. It may require surgical evacuation (vitrectomy) if persistent or associated with refractory increased intraocular pressure.

The underlying cause must be identified and treated.

Complications

- increased intraocular pressure, which may be refractory.

19.3 **The retina**

Investigation of retinal disease

Intravenous fluorescein angiography is a useful investigation in patients with retinal disease. Sodium fluorescein is injected into the antecubital vein and from there it is carried by the blood to the eye. When the retina is illuminated with blue light, the fluorescein in the vessels fluoresces and is recorded by a specialised camera. Fluorescein angiography reveals vascular occlusion, areas of reduced perfusion (hypoxaemia or ischaemia), or leakage of fluid from abnormal vessels, e.g. in proliferative diabetic retinopathy or disciform senile macular degeneration.

Retinal detachment

When the retina develops a hole, fluid from the vitreous humour seeps through this hole under the retina causing a retinal detachment (Fig. 132). Predisposing causes are:

- myopia
- previous cataract surgery
- trauma.

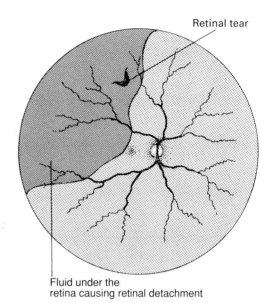

Retinal tear

Fluid under the retina causing retinal detachment

Fig. 132
Retinal detachment.

Clinical features

Clinical features include:

- history of floaters and/or flashing lights is common
- a 'shadow' coming over the field of vision
- rapid loss of vision.

If the detachment is large, ophthalmoscopy will reveal folds of retina sitting anteriorly in the vitreous cavity (Fig. 132).

Management

Surgical correction of the detachment is carried out using cryotherapy or laser treatment to seal the retinal hole. Gas may be injected into the vitreous cavity or small pieces of plastic may be sewn onto the outside of the globe to bring the retina into apposition with the choroid and to close the hole.

Age-related macular degeneration (ARMD)

This degenerative change at the central macula is a common cause of reduced vision, especially in the elderly population. It falls into two categories, dry macular degeneration (Fig. 133) and wet (or disciform) degeneration (Fig. 134).

Dry degeneration

Clinical features. The patient usually complains of gradual deterioration in vision, especially for reading. Ophthalmoscopy, through dilated pupils, demonstrates pigmentary mottling at the macular region (Fig. 133).

Management. No active treatment is available. The plan is to maximise the available vision by using a good light, magnifiers and big print. The patient may be eligible for partial sight or blind registration by a consultant ophthalmologist. The advantage of such registration is that the patient receives practical, social and educational support.

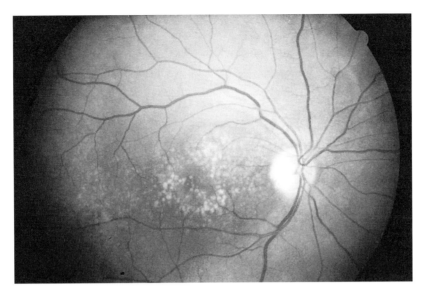

Fig. 133
Dry ARMD. There is evidence of retinal pigmentary disturbance at the macula.

Complications. Significant reduction in vision in extensive disease.

Wet degeneration (disciform)

In this more visually debilitating type of ARMD, blood vessels grow from the choroid under the retina at the macular region. They then leak or bleed.

Clinical features. The patient usually complains of distortion of images or sudden deterioration of vision (usually in one eye). A pale raised area is seen ophthalmoscopically at the macula, which may have some red or black haemorrhage around it (Fig. 134).

Management. In the early stages, laser treatment may be of benefit and fluorescein angiography defines the area for treatment. Vision should be maximised as for dry SMD.

Complications. The final visual outcome is usually poor. ARMD is the most common cause of blind registration in this country.

Retinal vascular occlusion

Occlusion of the retinal arteries or veins is a common cause of sudden visual loss.

Retinal artery occlusion

Arterial occlusion causes acute loss of vision. The most common cause is an embolus from a plaque of atheroma in the internal carotid artery.

Clinical features

Central retinal artery occlusion causes complete or almost complete painless loss of central and peripheral vision, which may be temporary (amaurosis fugax) or permanent (retinal artery occlusion). An embolus may be visible in an arteriole in either case. In patients with unrecovered disease, the retina becomes pale because of oedema, except at the fovea, which gives rise to the clin-

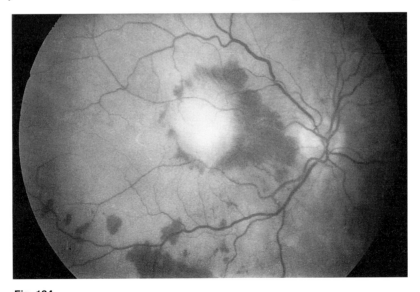

Fig. 134
Disciform ARMD. There is evidence of a pale raised lesion in the macular area with haemorrhage around the lesion. Some of this haemorrhage has spread inferiorly.

ical appearance of a cherry red spot at the macula. The vision does not improve.

The effect of occlusion of a branch artery depends on the area supplied by the vessel, but there is usually profound loss of central vision.

Diagnosis

The diagnosis is usually clinical but may be confirmed by intravenous fluorescein angiography (see Fig. 136B). The cardiovascular system must be examined for carotid bruits, valvular disease and atrial fibrillation.

Management

No treatment is effective in restoring visual function. The patient must be investigated to find a source for emboli. Low-dose aspirin may protect from further occlusions.

Retinal vein occlusion

Visual loss in retinal venous occlusion is not usually as profound as in retinal artery occlusions. Branch retinal venous occlusions are more common than central vein occlusions (see Fig. 136B).

The most important cause is hypertension. Diabetics have increased risk. Other causes include increased blood viscosity, e.g. from polycythaemia and multiple myeloma.

Clinical features

The patient develops sudden reduction of vision. The most striking feature of venous occlusion is multiple flame-shaped haemorrhages in the area of retina drained by the vessel (Fig. 135).

Management

Any associated systemic disease must be identified and treated. Fluorescein angiography (Fig. 136) is used to detect ischaemia, which can be treated with laser photocoagulation.

Complications. The most important complication is proliferative retinopathy resulting from the retinal ischaemia, which may give rise to vitreous haemorrhage and rubeotic glaucoma.

Diabetic retinopathy

Diabetic retinopathy is the most common cause of blindness in the working population. Therefore, diabetics must be screened regularly for retinopathy in order that treatment may be given early to prevent visual loss.

Classification

Diabetic retinopathy is usually categorised as:

- background retinopathy
- pre-proliferative retinopathy
- proliferative retinopathy
- maculopathy.

Clinical features

Background retinopathy. This is characterised by scattered dot haemorrhages and hard yellow exudates. The vision is normal.

Preproliferative retinopathy. This is characterised by cotton wool spots, blot haemorrhages and irregular dilatation of the retinal veins (venous beading). These findings indicate retinal ischaemia and, therefore, an increased risk of developing proliferative changes. The vision is normal.

Proliferative retinopathy. The hallmark of proliferative retinopathy is new vessel formation. These fibrovascular outgrowths arise from retinal veins in response to retinal ischaemia caused by diabetic microvascular occlusion. The new vessels arise either at the optic disc or at other more peripheral sites (Fig. 137). These new vessels may bleed causing vitreous haemorrhage or cause fibrosis, which applies traction to the retina, causing a tractional retinal detachment. Without treatment, patients with new disc vessels have a 50% chance of blindness within 5 years. The vision is, however, normal in the early stages of proliferative retinopathy and with appropriate treatment remains good.

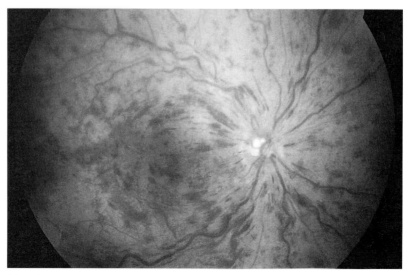

Fig. 135
Central retinal vein occlusion. Note the flame-shaped retinal haemorrhages and the dilated veins.

A

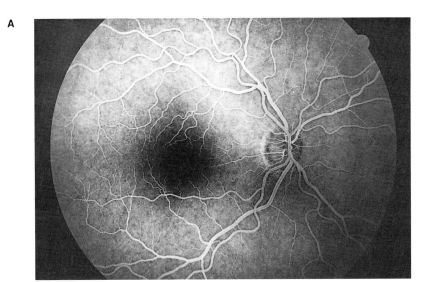

B

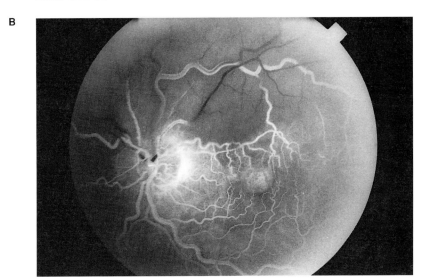

Fig. 136
Fluorescein angiography. **A.** This shows normal fluorescein angiography with background choroidal fluorescence and the arteries and veins showing up with no area of leakage. **B.** This is a fluorescein angiogram of a patient with a superior retinal branch vein occlusion. The inferior retina is vascularised normally but the blood supply to the superior area has been damaged with evidence of retrograde flow within the superior vein.

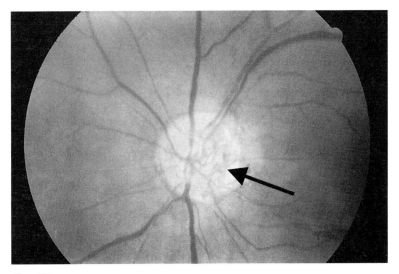

Fig. 137
Proliferative diabetic retinopathy. A leash of new vessels can be seen growing forward from the disc.

Maculopathy. When diabetic retinopathy affects the macular area, it is referred to as maculopathy. This may cause reduction in vision because of leakage of exudates or fluid from the capillaries or because of ischaemia. As the macula is a sensitive area for visual function, the vision usually deteriorates.

Diagnosis

Most types of retinopathy may be visualised with a direct ophthalmoscope. New vessels are best seen in red free light (using a green filter on the ophthalmoscope). If there is any doubt, neovascularisation can be confirmed on fluorescein angiography. The new vessels are abnormal and tend to leak dye.

Management

Background retinopathy does not require treatment. Patients with preproliferative retinopathy should be followed up frequently as this is a precursor to proliferative retinopathy. Proliferative retinopathy is treated with panretinal photocoagulation using an argon laser. Maculopathy may require laser treatment to preserve vision.

Complications

- vitreous haemorrhage
- retinal detachment
- secondary intractable glaucoma
- blindness.

Self-assessment: questions

Multiple choice questions

1. Choroidal malignant melanoma:
   a. Appears clinically as a pigmented raised lesion seen on fundoscopy
   b. Is the most common intraocular tumour
   c. Tends to metastasise to the lung
   d. Can be diagnosed by ultrasound scan of the eye
   e. Always requires extensive surgical excision

2. Acute anterior uveitis:
   a. Usually has a well-defined aetiology
   b. Is usually painful
   c. Commonly affects one eye
   d. Is associated with systemic toxoplasmosis
   e. Affects children with juvenile chronic arthritis

3. Features of background diabetic retinopathy are:
   a. Dot haemorrhages on the retina
   b. New vessel formation at the disc
   c. Irregular retinal veins
   d. Hard exudates
   e. Disc swelling

4. Venous occlusions of the retina:
   a. Are associated with carotid bruits
   b. May cause the development of a vitreous haemorrhage
   c. Often affect one branch of the vein
   d. May indicate an underlying problem, such as hypertension
   e. Are common in fit and healthy individuals

Case histories

History 1

A 35-year-old male presents with a red right eye. He says his vision is reduced and that it has been painful for the last 24 hours. There is no history of trauma and there has been no stickiness or discharge. He has a history of ankylosing spondylitis. Examination reveals a red eye with ciliary injection. The pupil is miosed. There is no corneal staining with fluorescein.

1. What is the most likely diagnosis?
2. What is the treatment?
3. Discuss the differential diagnosis (information from other sections is required to answer this question)

History 2

An 80-year-old lady attends as an emergency in the afternoon with sudden loss of vision in her right eye. She woke up that morning and was unable to see out of the eye. The vision in the right eye is hand movements (HM) and in the left is 6/9. The eyes are white and she has no pain. She suffers from angina, but otherwise is well.

1. What is the differential diagnosis?
2. Describe how each possible diagnosis can be confirmed and treated

Short notes

Write short notes on the following:

1. central retinal artery occlusion
2. dry macular degeneration
3. proliferative diabetic retinopathy

Self-assessment: answers

Multiple choice answers

1. a. **True.** Melanomas are usually raised pigmented lesions.
   b. **True.**
   c. **False.** Metastasis tends to be to the liver.
   d. **True.** Melanomas can be visualised with ultrasound.
   e. **False.** Management depends upon the size of the melanoma.

2. a. **False.** The underlying aetiology is rarely ascertained.
   b. **True.** It is usually painful.
   c. **True.** Acute anterior uveitis is usually unilateral.
   d. **False.** Posterior uveitis is caused by systemic toxoplasmosis.
   e. **True.** Children with juvenile chronic arthritis should be screened regularly for anterior segment inflammation.

3. a. **True.** Dot haemorrhages are a characteristic feature.
   b. **False.** New vessel formation is characteristic of proliferative retinopathy.
   c. **False.** Irregular retinal veins are present in preproliferative retinopathy.
   d. **True.** Hard exudates are characteristic.
   e. **False.**

4. a. **False.** Retinal arterial occlusions are associated with carotid disease.
   b. **True.** Retinal vein occlusions may lead to retinal ischaemia, which predisposes to new vessel formation which may, in turn, cause a vitreous haemorrhage.
   c. **True.** Small branch vein occlusions are common.
   d. **True.** Retinal vein occlusions are common in patients with hypertension.

   e. **False.** Fit healthy individuals rarely present with retinal venous occlusions.

Case history answers

History 1

1. The most likely diagnosis in this man is anterior uveitis (iritis). Factors that suggest this condition are that the man presents with a unilateral red eye associated with pain and reduced vision. He is young and has a history of anlkylosing spondylitis. Examination reveals ciliary injection but no fluorescein staining. The pupillary miosis is almost diagnostic of intraocular inflammation.
2. Treatment consists of topical steroids and cycloplegics.
3. The differential diagnosis of a red eye is: conjunctivitis, subconjunctival haemorrhage, episcleritis, corneal ulceration, uveitis, scleritis and acute-angle closure glaucoma. Table 2 lists the principal differences in these diagnoses.

History 2

1. An elderly lady with sudden loss of vision in one eye is most likely to have had an event affecting the vascular supply to the retina or optic nerve, i.e. central retinal vein occlusion, central retinal artery occlusion (or amaurosis fugax, if the loss of vision had been temporary) or anterior ischaemic optic neuropathy. The other possibility in this age group is disciform macular degeneration. Vitreous haemorrhage or retinal detachment are other causes of sudden loss of vision. The final possibility is that the lady has had a long-standing loss of vision in her right eye that she has just noticed because the vision in her left eye is normal. (See the gradual reduction in vision.) This often happens when the patient covers their better eye for some reason.

Table 2 Differential diagnosis of the red eye.

	Vision	Pain	Discharge	Area	Fluorescein staining	Pupil	Laterality
Conjunctivitis	Normal	Gritty	Sticky	Generalised	No	Normal	Both
Subconjunctival haemorrhage	Normal	No	No	Diffuse	No	Normal	One
Episcleritis	Normal	No	No	Interpalpebral	No	Normal	One
Corneal ulcer	Reduced	Yes	Yes/No	Limbal	Yes	Normal	One
Scleritis	Reduced	Yes	No	Variable	No	Normal	One/both
Uveitis	Reduced	Yes	No	Limbal	No	Small	One
Acute-angle closure glaucoma	Reduced	Yes	No	Diffuse	No	Mid-dilated	One (Second eye at risk)

2. Examination of the retina will provide most of the information in order to make a diagnosis. Central retinal vein occlusion will be recognised by the presence of diffuse flame-shaped haemorrhages over the retina, whereas the retina in a central retinal artery occlusion is pale with a cherry red spot at the macula and an embolus may be seen within the retinal arterial tree. The optic disc in anterior ischaemic optic neuropathy is swollen with haemorrhages around the nerve head. The macula in disciform degeneration is pale and raised, often with haemorrhage around the macular region. Retinal details are obscured by blood in cases of vitreous haemorrhage and folds of detached retina may be apparent in those with retinal detachment. Optic neuritis usually has no abnormal clinical findings except reduced vision and an afferent pupillary defect. It is important to ensure that this lady has no underlying treatable condition that has contributed to her loss of vision.

Short notes answers

1. Central retinal artery occlusions cause sudden loss of vision in one eye. The aetiology is usually an embolus from atheroma of the internal carotid arteries. Return of useful vision is uncommon and no treatment is possible. The patient should be investigated for carotid disease and treated appropriately with surgery or aspirin. Examination reveals a pale retina with a cherry red spot at the macula.

2. Dry macular degeneration is a common cause of progressive loss of vision in the elderly. The patients have particular problems with detailed visual tasks, such as reading. Examination of the macula reveals mottling of the pigment around the fovea. No active treatment is available, but the patient's vision should be maximised with the use of magnifiers, good reading lights and large print books. Some patients may require blind registration.

3. Proliferative diabetic retinopathy is diagnosed when new vessels are seen growing on the retina, usually at the optic disc, but may be at other sites. This may cause vitreous haemorrhage or lead to fibrosis which may lead to a retinal detachment. Treatment consists of retinal laser photocoagulation.

Strabismus

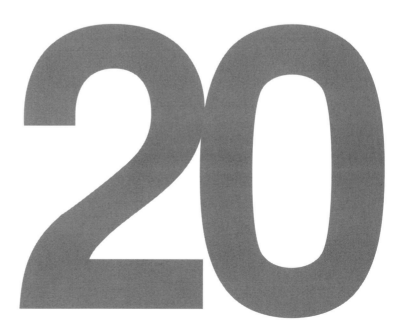

20.1 **Introduction**

Each eye has six extraocular muscles (the medial, lateral, inferior and superior rectus muscles and the inferior and superior obliques). The movements of each eye are finely coordinated with those of the opposite eye, so that both eyes normally function as one unit when fixating an object of interest in different fields of gaze. When the eyes become misaligned so that the visual axis of one eye is not directed to the same fixation point as the other, then a squint, or strabismus, is present.

Classification of squints:

- concomitant
    - convergent (esotropia) (Fig. 138A)
    - divergent (exotropia) (Fig. 138B)
    - vertical (hyper/hypotropia) (Fig. 138C)
- incomitant squints.

A concomitant squint is one that stays the same size no matter in which direction the patient looks and the patient has a full range of eye movements, whereas an incomitant one varies in size depending on the direction of gaze and there is evidence of weakness or tightness of one or more of the extraocular muscles. This distinction is important as it has implications regarding underlying aetiology, which is important in terms of investigation and management.

Incomitant squints are associated with:

- nerve palsies
- dysthyroid eye disease
- myasthenia gravis
- trauma.

20.2 **Concomitant squints**

Concomitant squints are common, and up to 5% of all children have such squints, the majority of which are convergent. Virtually all squints presenting in childhood are concomitant. Such squints are caused by an anomaly of the developing ocular motility system with no underlying organic disease. It is important to be able to identify squints in children, as if left untreated, they may result in poor vision in one eye (amblyopia).

Convergent squint (esotropia)

There is a strong association between hypermetropia (long-sightedness) and childhood esotropia.

This type of squint usually becomes evident at the age of about 18 months to $3\frac{1}{2}$ years, when the child's near reflex (i.e. the ability to converge and focus on a near object) is developing, so that the eyes tend to over-converge when trying to focus on a near object.

Clinical features
One eye turns inwards (Fig. 138A), which is confirmed

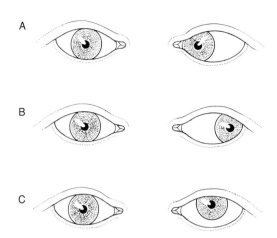

Fig. 138
Squints. **A.** Left esotropia. **B.** Left exotropia. **C.** Left hypertropia.

by the cover test. This eye commonly becomes amblyopic without treatment. The eye movements are full.

The squint may start as intermittent but becomes constant with time. There are usually no symptoms (such as double vision) as the patient develops suppression of the squinting eye.

Management
In this age group, any child with a squint should be tested for glasses (refracted), and any correction given to see if this improves or alters the angle of squint. If there is amblyopia (see below) this should be treated by patching the better eye. In patients whose vision is not corrected with spectacles, surgery is usually required.

Complications
The main complication of childhood squint is the development of amblyopia. Strabismic amblyopia is a condition in which there is a reduction in vision in one eye because it squints. Treatment of amblyopia consists of patching the other non-amblyopic eye for several hours each day to stimulate visually the amblyopic eye and, therefore, to assist its normal visual development. Any spectacle correction should be worn when patching is being carried out. Patching is only effective during the period of visual maturation (i.e. up to 8 years of age).

Pseudo-esotropia

Infants and small children often *appear* to have convergent squints when, in fact, their eyes are straight. This is because children's faces have wide nasal bridges and prominent epicanthal folds, which make them appear convergent. The cover test is used to confirm that there is no squint.

Divergent squint (exotropia)

Divergent squints are much rarer in children than convergent ones. The age of onset of this type of squint is from the very young infant to 5–6 years of age. The aetiology is unknown.

Clinical features

One eye tends to turn outwards (Fig. 138B), especially when looking in the distance. It often commences as an intermittent squint, but this becomes constant with time. The child tends to close one eye when looking in the distance. There is a full range of extraocular movements with no refractive error and no double vision.

Management

Surgery consists of weakening the lateral rectus muscle and/or strengthening the medial rectus to move the eye into a more central position.

20.3 Incomitant squints

This type of squint is usually caused by pathology of the nerve supply to the extraocular muscles or of the muscles themselves.

Incomitant squints may appear in children or adults. All children with squints should be examined with care to ensure that they do not have an incomitant squint. The features of incomitant squint depend on which muscles or nerves are affected. The presentation is usually of acute double vision.

Motor nerve palsies

The motor nerves to the extraocular muscles may be affected by a variety of disease processes such as:

- microvascular disease (in association with hypertension, diabetes or atherosclerosis)
- demyelination
- intracranial aneurysms
- infection (e.g. herpes zoster, meningitis)
- trauma
- intracranial neoplasms.

Clinical features

The features depend on the affected nerve.

Third nerve palsy. All muscles except the lateral rectus and superior oblique are innervated by the third (oculomotor) nerve. Features of a third nerve palsy include:

- divergent, hypotropic eye
- dilated, unreactive pupil
- ptosis (droopy upper lid).

In many patients, the condition is partial, either by sparing the pupil or lid or by leaving some movements partially or fully intact. A painful third nerve palsy must be considered as a **neurosurgical emergency** as this may be caused by enlargement of a posterior communicating artery aneurysm, which may be at risk of bleeding with catastrophic consequences.

Fourth nerve palsy. The fourth, or trochlear, nerve innervates the superior oblique muscle. The affected eye cannot look downwards fully while adducted (turned inwards) and patients notice diplopia in which the images are on top of each other (vertical diplopia) and at an angle to each other (torsional diplopia). To compensate for this the patients commonly tilt their heads away from the affected side (Fig. 139).

Sixth nerve palsy. Sixth (abducent) nerve palsy is the most common cranial nerve palsy. It causes an isolated lateral rectus weakness, which presents as double vision in which the images are side by side. The diplopia is maximal (i.e. the images are most widely separated) on looking towards the affected side and when looking in the distance (Fig. 140).

Management

The majority of nerve palsies improve spontaneously with time, usually a few months. They must be observed to allow time for improvement. During this time, the patient should be treated symptomatically to relieve any diplopia. This is done by patching one eye to occlude the second image or by sticking a plastic prism onto the glasses in front of one eye to allow the eyes to function together.

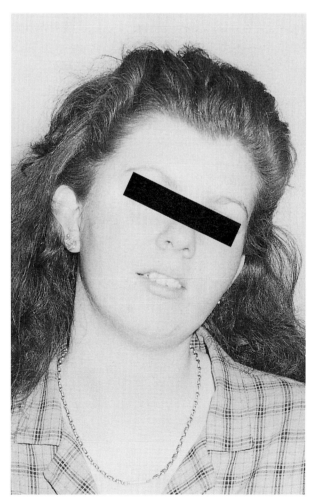

Fig. 139
Right fourth nerve palsy. Patients tilt their head away from the affected side.

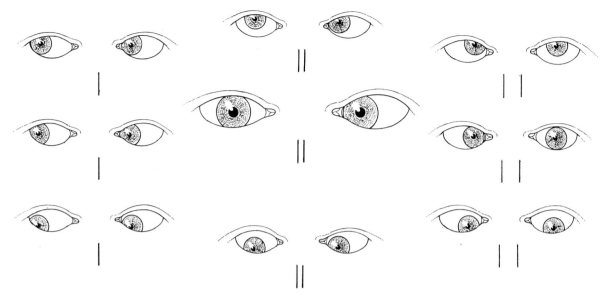

Fig. 140
Left sixth nerve palsy. A single image is seen on looking to the right, and the double images become progressively further apart when looking left.

In the long term, those that do not improve require definitive treatment to improve ocular alignment. In the majority of patients, this involves surgery to the affected muscles. In some patients, botulinum toxin injections may be used to weaken antagonist muscles. Toxin may be used in isolation or as a supplement to surgery.

Dysthyroid eye disease

Thyroid gland dysfunction can be associated with a disturbance of eye movements.

Clinical features

Patients often present with vertical or horizontal diplopia. In addition they usually have other features of dysthyroid eye disease, such as ocular discomfort and redness, lid retraction, lid lag and proptosis (Fig. 141). The abnormality of muscle function is not a weakness but a restriction caused by contraction of the affected muscles.

Patients with characteristic eye findings who have not previously been diagnosed as dysthyroid should have their thyroid function tested (thyroxine, triiodothyronine and thyroid-stimulating hormone). CT or MR scanning demonstrates thickened rectus muscles.

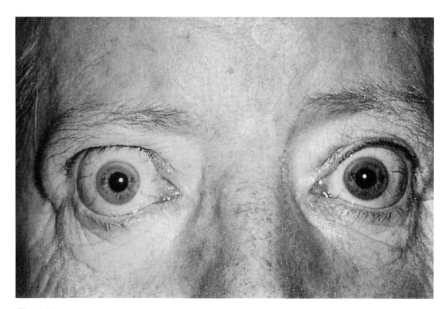

Fig. 141
Dysthyroid ophthalmopathy. Both upper and lower lids are retracted. Both eyes show proptosis.

Management

The underlying thyroid disorder should be treated. This, however, probably does not influence the clinical course of the eye disease. The condition runs an active course during which there may be continuing changes in the eye position, and during this time the patient should be kept comfortable with prisms or patches. After some months or years, this eventually stabilises and at this point the resultant ocular motility defects can be treated definitively, by operating to weaken (or recess) the restricted extraocular muscles.

Myasthenia gravis

Myasthenia gravis is an autoimmune condition in which neuromuscular transmission is affected by antibodies to the acetylcholine receptors.

Clinical features

The most common ocular sign is ptosis, although the patient may complain of diplopia, which may vary throughout the day and is characteristically worse at night. There is no pattern to the motility disturbance and it may simulate any nerve palsy.

Patients suspected of having myasthenia should have a tensilon (edrophonium) test. Acetylcholine receptor antibodies may be measured.

Management

Treatment is with pyridostigmine.

Self-assessment: questions

Multiple choice questions

1. Features of a sixth nerve palsy include:
   a. Reduced abduction of the affected eye
   b. Reduced vision in the affected eye
   c. Torsional diplopia
   d. Horizontal diplopia
   e. Maximum diplopia on looking away from the affected side

2. Features of an incomitant squint include:
   a. The same angle of squint in all positions of gaze
   b. Limitation of movement in one or more positions of gaze
   c. Diplopia
   d. Full correction of the angle of squint with spectacle wear
   e. Dizziness and unsteadiness

Short notes

Write short notes on:

1. dysthyroid eye disease
2. pseudo-esotropia
3. third nerve palsy

Essay question

Discuss the management of concomitant esotropia in children.

Viva questions

1. What is the medical term for squint?
2. What is the other term for a convergent squint?
3. What is the other term for a divergent squint?
4. What is the difference between a concomitant and an incomitant squint?
5. Give two causes of incomitant squint.
6. What are three possible causes of a nerve palsy?

Self-assessment: answers

Multiple choice answers

1. a. **True.** The sixth or abducent nerve innervates the lateral rectus muscle. This muscle abducts the eye.
   b. **False.**
   c. **False.**
   d. **True.**
   e. **False.** Patients suffer from maximum diplopia on looking towards the side of the lesion.

2. a. **False.** Incomitant squints vary in size of deviation depending on the direction of gaze.
   b. **True.**
   c. **True.** Patients often complain of diplopia, and this is usually the presenting complaint.
   d. **False.** Concomitant squints can be fully corrected with spectacles.
   e. **True.** This is due to weakness or reduced function of one or more extraocular muscles.

Short notes answers

1. Dysthyroid eye disease causes restriction of the extraocular rectus muscles, which may cause diplopia. The patient is usually hyperthyroid or has a history of hyperthyroidism. In addition, the eyes may be inflamed and irritable, with evidence of lid retraction and proptosis. The thyroid abnormality should be corrected and the patient's eye movements monitored until they become stable, when surgical correction may be considered.
2. Pseudo-esotropia is a condition in which a child appears to have a convergent squint because of the shape of their face, with the broad nose and epicanthal folds of childhood. The diagnosis is made on the basis of a normal cover test.
3. Third nerve palsy causes weakness of the medial, inferior and superior rectus and inferior oblique

muscles, so the eye is usually in a divergent and hypotropic position. In addition, the pupil is dilated and the upper lid droops. If the condition is painful it should be considered as a neurosurgical emergency as it may be caused by bleeding from an intracranial aneurysm.

Essay answer

Any squint should be confirmed with the cover test and the eye movements examined to ensure that it is concomitant. The vision should be checked using Kay's pictures or the Sheridan Gardiner test (depending on the age of the child) to find out if amblyopia is present. The child should be given any spectacle correction required and patching commenced if there is amblyopia. If glasses are not required or do not correct the squint, then surgery is needed to weaken the medial rectus and/or strengthen the lateral rectus muscles.

Viva answers

1. Strabismus.
2. Esotropia.
3. Exotropia.
4. In a concomitant squint, the patient has a full range of extraocular movements and the angle of the deviation is the same no matter in which direction the patient looks. There is evidence of muscle weakness or restriction in incomitant squints and the angle of deviation varies depending upon which direction the patient looks.
5. Nerve palsies, muscle disease or damage (trauma, dysthyroid eye disease, myasthenia gravis).
6. Any three of: microvascular disease, neoplasia, demyelination, aneurysms, infection or trauma.

Glaucoma

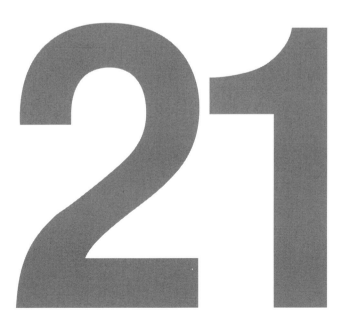

21.1 **Physiology**

The glaucomas are a group of conditions characterised by raised intraocular pressure (IOP), which causes damage to vision. The intraocular pressure is dependent on the rate of aqueous humour production and drainage. The normal range of intraocular pressure is 10–21 mmHg.

Aqueous fluid is produced by the ciliary body; it flows between the lens and the iris, through the pupil and into the anterior chamber. The fluid then drains through the trabecular meshwork, situated in the angle between the iris and the cornea, into the canal of Schlemm and thence into the venous circulation (Fig. 142). Glaucoma results from an abnormality in this system and is usually caused by reduced drainage of aqueous humour from the eye.

Outflow obstruction can occur in the presence of an open angle or a closed angle between the iris and the cornea.

Open angle. When the angle is open, the resistance to outflow is at the level of the trabecular meshwork. The aqueous humour cannot flow freely through the meshwork to reach the canal of Schlemm and the IOP increases gradually (Fig. 143).

Closed angle. The angle closes when the peripheral iris comes into contact with the cornea preventing the aqueous fluid reaching the trabecular meshwork (Fig. 144).

21.2 **Primary glaucoma**

Primary open-angle glaucoma

Primary open-angle glaucoma is usually a bilateral condition in which a gradual increase in IOP causes damage to the optic nerve head, which results in visual field loss. It is more common with increased age. There is a familial tendency, with 10% of first-degree relatives developing the disease.

The aetiology of resistance to aqueous outflow at the level of the trabecular meshwork is unknown.

Clinical features
The onset is insidious and the patient is usually asymptomatic until very late in the disease, when there is marked visual field loss. For this reason, all patients attending an optician for spectacles require screening for glaucoma. First-degree relatives of glaucoma patients require particular attention.

Diagnosis
The diagnosis of primary open-angle glaucoma is made on the basis of:

* raised intraocular pressure
* optic disc cupping (Fig. 145)
* visual field loss in the presence of an open anterior chamber drainage angle.

The intraocular pressure must be measured by an ophthalmologist. On ophthalmoscopy, the optic disc is seen to be cupped. The fields of vision need to be evaluated using computerised perimetry as the defects may be subtle in the early phase when treatment is most valuable. The typical field loss of glaucoma is an arcuate defect (scotoma) or nerve fibre bundle defect (Fig. 146). The central portion of the visual field is unaffected initially and the patient retains good visual acuity until late in the disease. Eventually the central portion of the field is lost and the patient becomes blind.

Management
Once visual field has been lost it is impossible to regain it; therefore, the aim of treatment is to lower the intraocular pressure in order to prevent optic nerve damage. Treatment is either medical, with laser or surgical.

Medical treatment takes the form of topically applied drops:

* beta-blockers (e.g. timolol) are usually the first line of treatment; they are instilled twice a day and have virtually no ocular side effects. It is important to

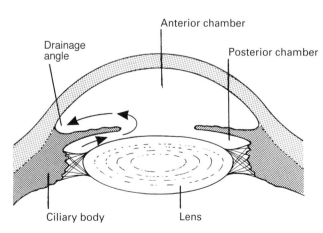

Fig. 142
Aqueous production, flow and drainage.

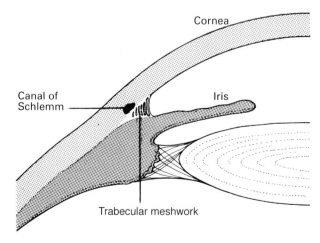

Fig. 143
Open angle. Blockage is at the level of the trabecular meshwork.

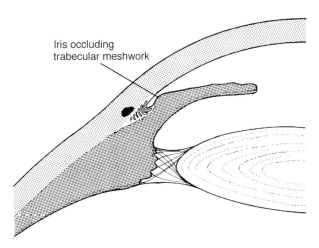

Fig. 144
Closed angle. Aqueous has no access to the angle structures as the iris lies against the cornea.

remember that patients with asthma or obstructive airways disease should not be given beta-blockers even topically
- topical adrenaline or adrenaline derivatives are also used twice a day but can cause pupil dilation
- topical parasympathomimetics (e.g. pilocarpine); they can cause headache and pupil constriction, which may reduce the vision, especially if cataract is present. These drops need to be instilled four times a day (which some people find inconvenient)
- topical carbonic anhydrase inhibitors are also effective
- new antiglaucoma drugs
- systemic carbonic anhydrase inhibitors (e.g. acetozolamide) reduce aqueous fluid formation but are rarely used as they have significant side effects. In patients where the IOP is poorly controlled, they may be used in combination with topical treatment in those who are unsuitable for, or are waiting for, surgery or laser treatment.

Laser treatment. Laser trabeculoplasty involves applying argon laser burns to the trabecular meshwork in order to improve the outflow. The long-term results of this form of treatment remain uncertain.

Surgical treatment. Surgery, or 'trabeculectomy', increases the outflow of aqueous fluid. A fistula is created surgically to allow a drainage of aqueous fluid into the sub-conjunctival space, bypassing the drainage angle and lowering the pressure. Trabeculectomy has a high success rate but may be complicated by intraocular infection, intraocular haemorrhage and premature cataract formation.

Complications
Untreated open-angle glaucoma may progress to blindness.

Ocular hypertension

In some patients the IOP is elevated but there is no evidence of optic disc cupping or typical field defects. This is termed 'ocular hypertension'. The patient does not require any treatment, although they should be

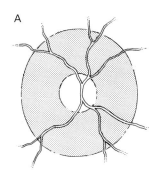

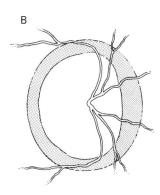

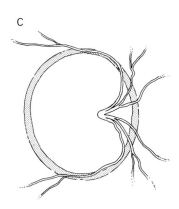

Fig. 145
Optic disc. **A.** Normal optic disc with small central cup. **B.** Early glaucomatous cupping with extension of the cup vertically. **C.** Advanced glaucomatous cupping.

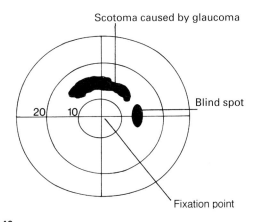

Fig. 146
Pattern of field loss in early open-angle glaucoma, in arcuate scotoma (or nerve fibre bundle defect).

reviewed regularly as they are at increased risk of developing glaucoma (i.e. developing disc cupping and field defects).

Low-tension glaucoma

A group of patients show evidence of disc damage and glaucomatous field defects, despite consistently normal pressures (< 21 mmHg). The cause of their sensitivity to low pressures is unknown, although there is an association with arterial disease. The diagnosis of low tension glaucoma is made by exclusion after intracranial causes of visual field loss have been excluded.

Primary angle-closure glaucoma

In contrast to the insidious onset of open-angle glaucoma, this type of glaucoma presents as an acute, painful red eye with poor vision. Although bilateral, it rarely affects both eyes at the same time; it is, therefore, important to treat the fellow eye prophylactically to prevent it developing a full-blown attack.

The primary abnormality in this condition is that the aqueous fluid is unable to flow from the posterior chamber into the anterior chamber. This is because of an increased resistance to the flow of aqueous fluid between the lens and the iris at the pupil, known as 'pupil block'. This occurs when the pupil is mid-dilated. The aqueous fluid becomes trapped in the posterior chamber, pushing the iris forwards and making the anterior chamber very shallow; this occludes the trabecular meshwork with the peripheral iris so that the angle closes (Fig. 147). The symptoms are caused by the resultant rapid increase in the intraocular pressure. Primary angle closure is more common in people with a hypermetropic spectacle error (i.e. have small eyes).

Clinical features

The patient presents with an extremely painful red eye that may be associated with nausea and vomiting. The eye is diffusely red, there is no discharge, the cornea is cloudy, the pupil is mid-dilated and unreactive to light. There is profound visual loss.

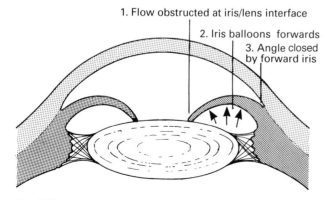

1. Flow obstructed at iris/lens interface
2. Iris balloons forwards
3. Angle closed by forward iris

Fig. 147
Sequence of events in primary closed angle glaucoma.

Prior to the acute episode, the patient may give a history of intermittent episodes of ocular pain and seeing haloes round lights, especially in the evenings. These attacks resolve spontaneously but should alert the doctor to the risk of acute angle-closure glaucoma.

The diagnosis is made on the basis of a typical history, in association with a shallow anterior chamber, extremely high IOP and a pupil that is mid-dilated and unreactive to light. Digital pressure (i.e. simply pressing on the eye) reveals a brick hard eye.

Management

The immediate treatment is to lower the pressure as quickly as possible using intravenous carbonic anhydrase inhibitors and to reverse the attack by breaking the pupil block using topical pilocarpine which mioses the pupil. Long-term treatment will involve both eyes as the condition is bilateral and both eyes will require surgery.

The affected eye. If the acute attack is reversed medically then a peripheral iridectomy is carried out. A peripheral iridectomy is a small hole created in the peripheral iris that allows aqueous fluid to flow directly from the posterior chamber into the anterior chamber without passing through the pupil, thus preventing a further attack. This can be performed surgically, but more commonly it is achieved using a laser (laser iridotomy). This is carried out on an out-patient basis and does not involve surgery to the eye. If the acute attack is not reversed using medical treatment, then a trabeculectomy is required (see above).

The fellow eye. In all cases, the other eye is at high risk of developing an acute attack of angle closure and a peripheral iridectomy is carried out prophylactically.

Complications. If the acute attack continues unabated, the eye becomes permanently blind.

21.3 Secondary glaucoma

Glaucoma may occur secondary to a number of ocular conditions that reduce outflow of aqueous fluid from the eye.

- trauma, causing damage to the drainage angle or secondary to hyphaema
- uveitis, usually through inflammation and swelling of the trabecular meshwork
- mature cataract: the lens swells up and the iris is pushed forwards to close the angle
- new vessel formation caused by ischaemia may grow into the angle of the eye and this may fibrose and close the angle (rubeosis)
- topical steroid treatment: some people develop raised IOP when using topical steroids, they are known as 'steroid responders'
- following intraocular surgery, usually because of postoperative inflammation.

Management

In these conditions, treatment is aimed at the primary disorder as well as control of the intraocular pressure.

21.4 Congenital glaucoma

Primary congenital glaucoma is an extremely rare disease that is usually bilateral owing to abnormal development of the anterior chamber drainage angle.

Clinical features

In the early stages, the cornea becomes oedematous, which causes photophobia and watering of the eye.

Affected infants commonly rub their eyes. In untreated or poorly controlled disease, the eye becomes enlarged (end-stage disease is called buphthalmos, or ox eye).

Management

If the diagnosis is suspected, the child should be examined under anaesthetic and the intraocular pressure measured. Treatment is surgical. The drainage angle is opened (goniotomy). Alternatively a trabeculectomy may be required.

Complications. Without rapid control of the pressure, the child becomes blind.

Self-assessment: questions

Multiple choice questions

1. Primary open-angle glaucoma:
   a. Causes severe pain
   b. Is associated with a normal visual field
   c. Has a familial tendency
   d. Causes disc cupping
   e. May be treated by peripheral iridectomy

2. The following are characteristics of primary angle-closure glaucoma:
   a. Myopic refractive error
   b. Severe ocular pain
   c. Mid-dilated unreactive pupil
   d. Normal vision
   e. Nausea and vomiting

3. Treatment of primary open-angle glaucoma may consist of:
   a. Topical beta-blockers
   b. Topical alpha and beta stimulants
   c. Topical parasympatheticolytics
   d. Retinal laser treatment
   e. Trabeculectomy

Essay question

What is the pathophysiology of acute angle-closure glaucoma? How does it present?

Short notes

Write short notes on:

1. ocular hypertension
2. congenital glaucoma
3. treatment of primary open-angle glaucoma

Viva questions

1. Give three ocular conditions which may predispose to secondary glaucoma.
2. What condition causes arcuate field loss and cupping of the optic disc, while the patient has normal intraocular pressures?
3. How would you treat an acute attack of angle-closure glaucoma?
4. What are the cardinal signs of primary open-angle glaucoma?

Self-assessment: answers

Multiple choice answers

1. a. **False.**
   b. **False.** It causes visual defects.
   c. **True.** Of first-degree relatives, 10% will develop the disease.
   d. **True.**
   e. **False.** Surgical treatment is trabeculectomy; it is angle-closure glaucoma that is treated by peripheral iridectomy.

2. a. **False.** Primary angle-closure glaucoma is associated with a hypermetropic spectacle error, not a myopic one.
   b. **True.** The patient has a red painful eye.
   c. **True.** One of the most important features of acute angle-closure glaucoma, which differentiates it from other causes of a red painful eye, is the presence of a mid-dilated, unreactive pupil.
   d. **False.** The vision is reduced during an attack of acute angle-closure.
   e. **True.** The patient feels generally unwell, often with nausea and vomiting.

3. a. **True.** Topical beta-blockers are often the first line of management in patients who have no contradindications. They are well tolerated , have no effect on pupil size and are only used twice a day.
   b. **True.** Topical alpha and beta stimulants, such as insulin, are used. Another type of drug which may be used topically is a parasympathetico-mimetic, such as pilocarpine.
   c. **False.**
   d. **False.**
   e. **True.** This may be required in some patients.

Essay answer

Acute angle-closure glaucoma occurs when the lens/iris contact reaches a critical area in susceptible eyes, such that the flow of aqueous humour from the posterior chamber through the pupil into the anterior chamber becomes interrupted. This situation is known as pupil block. The iris becomes pushed forward by the build up of aqueous in the posterior chamber and the drainage angle becomes closed off by this bowing forward of the iris. Susceptible eyes are those which are hypermetropic and those that have a large lens, i.e. those of older people.

This usually presents as a red, painful eye with reduced vision. The patient may also have systemic upset, such as nausea and vomiting and severe headache. Examination reveals reduced vision in the affected eye (usually 6/60 or less), and a diffusely injected eye with corneal cloudiness due to oedema. The anterior chamber appears shallow and the *pupil is fixed and mid-dilated.* The eye feels brick hard to touch. This is usually a unilateral presentation, although the other eye is at increased risk of developing the same problem.

Short notes answers

1. Ocular hypertension is a condition where the intraocular pressure is elevated, but there is no evidence of any optic disc cupping and the fields of vision are full. The patient should be observed and no treatment is required.

2. Congenital glaucoma is a rare condition that, if left untreated, progresses to blindness in affected children. The cause is abnormal development of the drainage angle. The clinical signs are watering of the eyes and photophobia. If the condition advances, the eyes become enlarged. Examination under anaesthetic is required to measure accurately the intraocular pressure in children. Surgery is the definitive treatment.

3. Primary open-angle glaucoma can be treated by medical treatment, laser treatment or surgery. Medical treatment involves the instillation of drops, either beta-blockers, sympathomimetics or parasympathols. Laser treatment improves the outflow of aqueous fluid. Surgical treatment takes the form of a trabeculectomy.

Viva answers

1. Glaucoma may be secondary to trauma, surgery, uveitis, mature cataract, topical steroid treatment or ocular ischaemia.
2. Low-tension glaucoma.
3. Intravenous acetazolamide and topical pilocarpine to reduce IOP. Peripheral iridotomy to both eyes, although the affected eye may require a trabeculectomy.
4. Increased intraocular pressure, disc cupping and field loss.

Ocular injuries

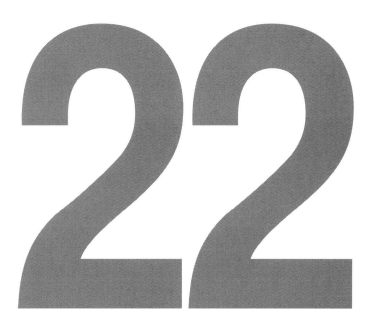

22.1 Introduction

Injuries to the eye are an important cause of ocular morbidity and visual impairment. The majority occur in young men. Most are superficial, with less than 30% being considered sight-threatening. The common causes are sport and leisure activities, accidents in the workplace or home, assaults and road traffic accidents.

Prevention of injuries

The treatment of eye injuries is expensive and in many cases disappointing; therefore, the best method of reducing this burden is prevention. Although effective protective eyewear is available for most high-risk activities, such as sports and work, unfortunately it is frequently not worn properly.

22.2 Blunt injuries

Blunt injuries are the most common type of eye injury. They are caused by a direct blow to the eye and surrounding tissues by an object such as a fist or a ball. Rapidly moving objects are more damaging than those moving at a lower velocity, even if they are larger and heavier.

Minor blunt injuries cause bruising of the eyelids and superficial ocular structures. The cornea epithelium may also be damaged by a blow.

If the eye is struck hard enough, the globe flattens anteroposteriorly and becomes stretched equatorially (Fig. 148); thus intraocular structures are damaged by a combination of contusional and tearing forces. No penetration takes

place although in severe cases rupture of the periorbital skin or eyeball may occur. The rapid increase in intraorbital pressure may cause a 'blow-out fracture' of the floor of the orbit, in which the orbital rim remains intact (Fig. 149), but the floor of the orbit fractures into the maxillary antrum.

Clinical features

Common features of blunt ocular trauma include:

- periorbital haematoma (black eye)
- blow-out fracture, causing double vision, enophthalmos and infraorbital anaesthesia
- subconjunctival haemorrhage, or diffuse bleeding under the conjunctiva
- corneal abrasion: an acutely painful injury that can be detected by instilling fluorescein drops into the conjunctival sac and the abraded area will stain bright green when viewed with a blue light
- hyphaema (blood in the anterior chamber) (Fig. 150): this indicates that the eye has suffered a significant injury with damage to the intraocular structures; the eye is usually acutely painful especially if the intraocular pressure is elevated, which is a common effect of blood in the eye
- rare, sight-threatening effects include retinal holes, choroidal tear and rupture of the globe.

Management

Black eyes and subconjunctival haemorrhages settle spontaneously over a few days without any treatment. Corneal abrasions are treated with antibiotic ointment and firm padding. Blow-out fractures only require surgical intervention if double vision persists. In cases of intraocular damage, full examination of the eye may not be possible until bleeding has settled and the eye is stable, which may be 3–4 weeks after the injury. Patients may require hospital admission and complications such as increased intraocular pressure and rebleeding (secondary hyphaema) are treated medically, although secondary hyphaemas may require to be surgically evacuated. Examination should include the peripheral retina for tears and an assessment of the drainage angle.

Early complications:

- raised intraocular pressure
- uveitis
- rebleeding of hyphaemas.

Long-term complications:

- recurrent corneal erosions
- premature cataract
- glaucoma
- retinal detachment.

22.2 Small flying particles

Low-velocity foreign material tends to lodge on the cornea as a corneal foreign body (CFB) or under the lid

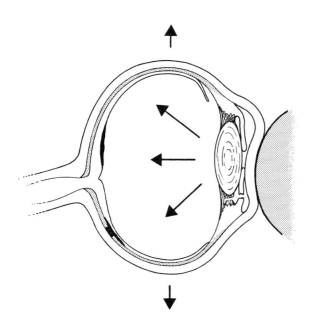

Fig. 148
When the eye is struck, it is deformed and intraocular structures are damaged.

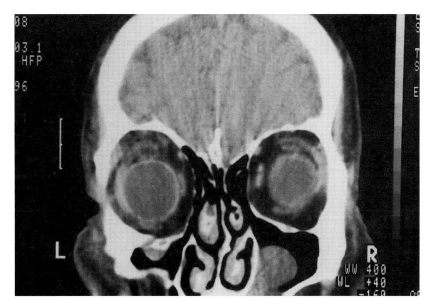

Fig. 149
A 'blow-out' fracture of the right orbit, shown on CT scan. The orbit is expanded and there is evidence of a prolapse of tissue into the maxillary antrum through the orbital floor (the tear-drop sign).

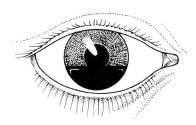

Fig. 150
Hyphaema.

as a subtarsal foreign body (STFB). High-velocity particles penetrate the globe to become intraocular foreign bodies (IOFB). Any injury that may have been caused by a high-velocity small particle (e.g. hammering injuries) should be treated as a potentially penetrating IOFB until proved otherwise, i.e. an X-ray of the eye should be performed or an experienced opthalmologist's opinion sought before discounting this diagnosis.

Clinical features
Superficial FBs cause a significant amount of pain, watering, redness and photophobia. Paradoxically, intraocular foreign material may be less painful and the symptoms are frequently minor.

Corneal foreign bodies can usually be seen on close inspection of the cornea and staining with fluorescein helps to demarcate the area. STFBs can be seen when the upper eyelid is everted (Fig. 116, p. 161).

IOFBs may be difficult to see on examination, although the pupil may be irregular.

Management
Corneal foreign bodies can be removed by a small cotton tip or a sharp needle (under magnification after the instillation of topical anaesthetic). An STFB can be swept off the inside of the lid after everting the lid with a cotton tip. If there is any epithelial damage from the superficial FB, then topical antibiotic agents and a firm pad are applied.

IOFBs require surgical removal. This may involve loss of the lens, iris or vitreous humour if they are damaged by the injury.

Complications
The damaged epithelium of the cornea may not heal satisfactorily after a CFB or an STFB, leading to a recurrent corneal erosion, a painful condition caused by recurrent breakdown of a tiny area of the epithelial surface.

The long-term effects of an IOFB depend on the degree of intraocular damage and the type and size of material that penetrated the eye. Organic material may rapidly lead to suppuration of the intraocular contents, and metallic foreign bodies oxidise and combine with the intraocular proteins (siderosis) if not removed in the early period.

22.3 Large sharp objects

Injuries caused by large sharp objects may penetrate the eye.

Clinical features
The clinical features depend on the extent of the injury, ranging from superficial damage to the lids and eye to full ocular penetration with globe disruption.

Ocular penetrations may be manifest as an irregular pupil because the iris plugs the wound to prevent the loss of intraocular contents (Fig. 151); or the eyes may be softer than normal. The vision is usually reduced.

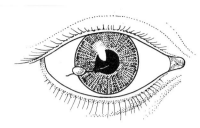

Fig. 151
Penetrating injury. A corneal laceration is seen, with the iris plugging the wound.

One should aways be suspicious that full thickness lid lacerations may involve the underlying sclera and retina.

Management
Lid lacerations, like any facial injuries, require careful skin closure. However, as the lacrimal drainage apparatus is situated at the medial aspect of the lid (Fig. 120, p. 166), injuries in this area may require specialist evaluation and treatment.

A primary repair for globe penetration should be performed urgently. Multiple surgical procedures may subsequently be required for the optimum result.

Complications
* Corneal scarring
* Cataract
* Endophthalmitis
* Sympathetic ophthalmia is a very rare granulomatous inflammation that affects both eyes after a penetrating injury to one eye. The injured (exciting) eye sets up this response in itself as well as in the other (sympathising) eye. This usually occurs within 3 months of the injury. Removal of the injured eye before the sympathetic response starts prevents the onset of the condition; once established, removal of the exciting eye does not help. The response to steroids and immunosuppressants is usually favourable. Removal of an injured eye should, therefore, not be considered purely on the grounds of the risk of sympathetic ophthalmia but be based on the visual potential of the eye.

22.4 Burns

Burns to the eye are divided into chemical or physical burns.

Chemical burns

Burns caused by acids or alkalis are a medical emergency. Alkalis denature proteins and their burns tend to be more extensive and penetrating than acid burns.

Clinical features
Patients with chemical burns to the eye are in severe pain. There may be lid swelling, oedema of the conjunctiva, corneal and conjunctival epithelial loss, uveitis, raised intraocular pressure, corneal melting, cataract and peripheral retinal damage.

Management
Any patient with a history of a chemical being splashed into the eyes must be treated with immediate copious irrigation of the affected eyes with water or normal saline. Any particulate material (e.g. lime) should be looked for and removed from the fornices or subtarsal areas urgently. There should be no delay to obtain a careful history or to examine the eyes.

Once thorough irrigation has been completed (20–30 minutes), the extent of damage may be evaluated. Corneal and conjunctival epithelium may be totally lost. In addition, the blood vessels may be destroyed leading to areas of scleral ischaemia and the cornea may be rendered opaque.

Complications

* severe corneal and conjunctival scarring
* raised intraocular pressure
* cataract
* necrosis of sclera
* ultimately, perforation of the eye with loss of useful vision.

Physical burns

Physical burns can be caused by:

* thermal energy
* ultraviolet (UV)
* shorter wave radiation (e.g. radiotherapy).

Thermal burns do not usually involve the globe itself, as reflex blinking provides natural protection.

UV radiation is absorbed by the corneal epithelium which causes the conditions of snow blindness or welding flash burns.

Iatrogenic ocular damage may occur from radiation used to treat head and neck cancers and may not become evident until many years later. It usually manifests as premature cataract and radiation retinal vasculitis.

Self-assessment: questions

Multiple choice questions

1. An intraocular foreign body (IOFB):
   a. Can usually be seen on clinical examination
   b. Should be suspected in patients with high-velocity injuries
   c. Is usually very painful
   d. Needs urgent surgical removal
   e. Can cause significant intraocular damage

2. Alkali burns of the eye:
   a. Are potentially more serious than acid burns
   b. May cause secondary raised intraocular pressure
   c. Are a cause of entropion
   d. Are a medical emergency
   e. Can cause necrosis of the sclera

3. Late complications of blunt trauma include:
   a. Raised intraocular pressure
   b. Retinal detachment
   c. Retinal vein occlusion
   d. Cataract
   e. Sympathetic ophthalmia

Case history

> A 28-year-old joiner who was hammering nails into a wooden stake without any ocular protection presents to the casualty department, having felt something going into his right eye:

1. What is the likely injury?
2. How would you assess him?
3. What management may be required?

Essay question

What happens to the eye when it it struck by a blunt object and what injuries can this cause to the eye?

Short notes

Write short notes on:

1. sympathetic ophthalmia
2. the immediate management of a chemical burn to the eye
3. hyphaema
4. blow-out fracture

Self-assessment: answers

Multiple choice answers

1. a. **False.** IOFBs are often virtually painless and may easily be missed on clinical examination.
   b. **True.** Any person who presents with an eye injury which has been caused by a high-velocity flying particle must be suspected as having an IOFB. Hammering injuries are common causes of IOFBs, as the head of a hammer becomes brittle with use and small pieces tend to fly off and enter the eye.
   c. **False.** IOFBs are often virtually painless.
   d. **True.** They must be removed as soon as is possible, as they may cause further toxic damage inside the eye.
   e. **True.** IOFBs can cause damage as they enter the eye.

2. a. **True.** Alkali burns tend to be more extensive and penetrating.
   b. **True.**
   c. **True.** They may cause cicatricial changes of the conjunctiva which results in inturning of the eyelid (entropion).
   d. **True.** Alkali burns are potentially serious sight-threatening injuries which need to be treated urgently.
   e. **True.**

3. a. **True.** Blood inside the eye may block the trabecular meshwork and lead to raised intraocular pressure.
   b. **True.** Any tear in the peripheral retina at the time of injury will predispose to a retinal detachment.
   c. **False.**
   d. **True.** The metabolism of the lens may be damaged leading to premature lens opacities.
   e. **False.** Sympathetic ophthalmia is a complication of penetrating trauma.

Case history answer

1. The most likely diagnosis is an intraocular foreign body (IOFB) injury caused by a small flying particle from the head of the hammer.
2. The vision should be measured. The pupil should be examined; it may be distorted if material has entered the eye. Any patient who has suffered an eye injury while hammering needs to have an IOFB excluded and, even if there are no clinical signs to support the diagnosis, an X-ray of the orbit should be taken. If there are any clinical signs of an IOFB or the X-ray confirms the presence of an IOFB, then the patient should be referred to an ophthalmologist.
3. The patient will require surgical removal of the foreign material to prevent long-term complications of retained metal. In addition surgery will repair

any intraocular structures damaged by the piece of penetrating material (e.g. corneal lacerations, lens damage, retinal tears).

Essay answer

When the eye is struck by a blunt object it suffers a contusional type of injury. Mild injuries cause bruising to the periorbital tissues (periorbital haematoma or black-eye), bleeding under the conjunctiva (sub-conjunctival haemorrhage) or remove the epithelium from the cornea (corneal abrasion). More severe trauma results in deformation of the globe itself and this causes damage to the intraocular structures by a combination of stretching and contusional forces. This may result in bleeding inside the eye (hyphaema) or damage to the retina or choroid. The orbital floor may fracture in severe injuries (blow-out fracture).

Very severe injuries may result in rupture of the eye.

Short notes answers

1. Sympathetic ophthalmia is a very rare inflammatory condition that affects both eyes after a penetrating injury has taken place to one eye. This can be prevented by removing the injured eye shortly after the injury has taken place. However, the injured eye may retain some useful vision and the risk of sympathetic ophthalmia is so low that traumatised eyes should not be removed prophylactically unless there is no prospect of any visual prognosis in that eye. Treatment is of sympathetic ophthalmia with systemic steroids and antimetabolites.
2. The immediate management of a chemical burn involves rapid and copious irrigation of the affected eye(s) with water or saline. Any particulate matter should be removed. Early assessment should involve identifying areas of epithelial loss and ischaemia.
3. A hyphaema is the presence of blood inside the anterior chamber. This is usually visible as a level of blood at the bottom of the chamber. It is the hallmark of significant intraocular damage and indicates that the eye should be examined for other damage (e.g. retinal tears). There is a risk of secondary raised intraocular pressure and the patient may need hospital admission.
4. A blow-out fracture involves the floor of the orbit, although the orbital rim remains intact. It is caused by a rapid rise in intraorbital pressure when the eye is struck by a blunt object and the contents of the inferior part of the orbit decompress into the maxillary antrum. The clinical features are of infraorbital anaesthesia, enophthalmos and diplopia. Surgical correction is only considered if the double vision is troublesome and persistent.

Neuro-ophthalmology

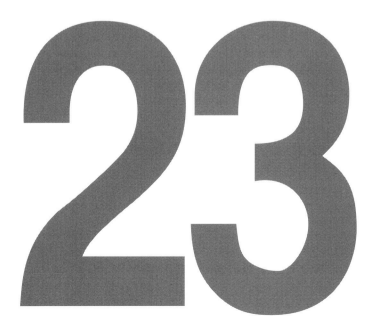

23.1 Introduction

Visual information from the eyes is transferred via the optic nerves, chiasm, optic tracts, lateral geniculate bodies and optic radiations to the occipital cortex for interpretation and integration. A number of pathological processes that may cause defects in the fields of vision can occur at any point along this pathway.

23.2 Optic nerve

The optic nerve is part of the central nervous system and, as such, can be involved in neurological diseases as well as diseases of the eye (e.g. glaucoma). In this section, conditions of the optic nerve considered are:

- optic neuritis
- anterior ischaemic optic neuropathy
- papilloedema
- optic atrophy.

Optic neuritis

This is an inflammation of the optic nerve, which usually occurs in adults aged 15–50 as a result of:

- demyelination
- viral infections
- idiopathic causes.

When the optic nerve head is involved this is termed papillitis and when the nerve behind the globe is affected it is called retrobulbar neuritis. These conditions have the same aetiology, management and implications; they simply involve slightly different areas of the optic nerve.

Clinical features

The main clinical features are:

- usually one eye affected
- reduction in vision over a few days with loss of colour vision (may be mild or severe, but the patient finds that bright red appears as a desaturated red or pink)
- pain when moving the eye, especially upwards
- gradual recovery of visual function over a period of 1–4 weeks
- further blurring of vision with exertion or increased heat (Uhtoff's phenomenon).

The only sign of optic neuritis may be an afferent pupillary defect (see below) in association with poor visual acuity. Patients with papillitis also have swelling of the optic nerve head. Field of vision testing demonstrates a central scotoma in the affected eye. The visual evoked response demonstrates increased latency.

Management

Management is simply observation and awaiting the recovery of vision.

Complications. In a small proportion of patients, the vision does not recover; in particular, the colour perception remains abnormal.

Anterior ischaemic optic neuropathy

Anterior ischaemic optic neuropathy represents an infarction of the optic nerve head, usually affecting patients over 60. It is caused by vascular disease. Two types are recognised:

- arteritic, giant cell arteritis
- atherosclerotic.

Clinical features

The clinical features of each type of anterior ischaemic optic neuropathy are similar:

- rapid, painless drop in vision usually total in the affected eye but may affect the upper or lower field only (altitudinal field defect, Fig. 152)
- vision usually significantly impaired
- disc swelling, with haemorrhages around the posterior pole
- no visual recovery.

It is important to differentiate between arteritic and atherosclerotic causes, as this has important implications regarding management.

Diagnosis

Diagnosis of the arteritic variety is made on the basis of the patient suffering from a systemic disorder consisting of general malaise, headaches, muscle tenderness and jaw claudication in the presence of an elevated ESR (usually > 100 mm/h) or elevated plasma viscosity. A temporal artery biopsy is indicated to establish the diagnosis unequivocally.

Those with the atherosclerotic type may have symptoms of generalised arteriopathic disease, such as angina or intermittent claudication.

Management

Systemic steroids are used in those with giant cell arteritis. High doses of systemic steroids must be commenced **immediately** to preserve the vision in the other eye. Steroid treatment may be required for many years. There is a 65% chance of the other eye being affected within 10 days.

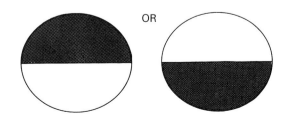

Fig. 152
Altitudinal field defect; loss of upper or lower field.

No effective treatment is available for atherosclerotic cases.

Complications

- the other eye becomes affected (almost invariably in those with temporal arteritis without treatment, and in approximately 30% of the others)
- generalised complications of vascular disease.

Papilloedema

This term refers to swelling of the optic nerve head caused by increased intracranial pressure. Intracranial space-occupying lesions and benign intracranial hypertension (pseudo-tumour cerebri) are the most common causes.

Clinical features

The main clinical features are:

- good visual function
- headaches, nausea and vomiting
- ophthalmoscopy reveals elevation of the optic disc, blurring of the disc margins, dilatation of the retinal veins and haemorrhages around the disc
- field of vision testing shows an enlarged blind spot.

Diagnosis

Intracranial imaging with CT or MR should reveal any intracranial mass. If this is negative, a lumbar puncture should be performed to measure the intracranial pressure.

Management

Neurosurgical decompression of any intracranial space-occupying lesion is required.

Optic atrophy

This is not a diagnosis but is a clinical sign that may result from a number of different disease processes that affect the optic nerve:

- optic neuritis
- ischaemic optic neuropathy
- chronic papilloedema
- optic nerve tumours
- optic nerve trauma
- ocular disease (e.g. glaucoma, retinal artery occlusion).

Clinical features

Reduction in visual acuity or field of vision is a usual clinical finding. The presenting complaint usually depends on the underlying cause. The optic disc is pale in appearance on ophthalmoscopy.

Management

Treat the underlying cause.

23.3 **Optic chiasm**

The optic chiasm is the area of the visual pathways where the visual pathways partially cross. The chiasm is situated just above the pituitary gland and enlarging adenomas of the pituitary, usually chromophobe or eosinophil, can lead to compression of the chiasm.

Clinical features

Patients with pituitary adenomas classically present with headache, hormonal disturbance and a bitemporal hemianopia (Fig. 153). CT scan of the pituitary region will usually reveal the underlying pathology.

Management

Neurosurgical decompression is required.

23.4 **Retro-chiasmal pathway**

The retro-chiasmal pathway includes the optic tract, optic radiation and the occipital cortex.

These postchiasmal optic pathways may be involved in:

- cerebrovascular accidents
- tumours
- infections (meningitis, cerebral abscesses).

These lesions cause defects in the visual field of both eyes and may also be responsible for other neurological deficits. The field defects depend on the area of the pathway that is affected, but postchiasmal lesions are always homonymous (i.e. affect the same side of the visual field in each eye) (Fig. 153).

Clinical features

The presentation may be part of a more generalised neurological disorder, e.g. a cerebrovascular accident or raised intracranial pressure. Visual fields should be tested to identify the site of the lesion.

Diagnosis

Intracranial imaging, using CT or, preferably, MRI, identifies the site and nature of the lesion.

Management

Visual field anomalies are usually irreversible, although if caused by pressure they may improve after neurosurgical intervention.

23.5 **The pupils**

Abnormalities of the pupils may reflect neurological disease. The afferent limb of the pupillary light reflex is via the retina, optic nerve, chiasm and optic tract. This passes to the third nerve nucleus and synapses there to

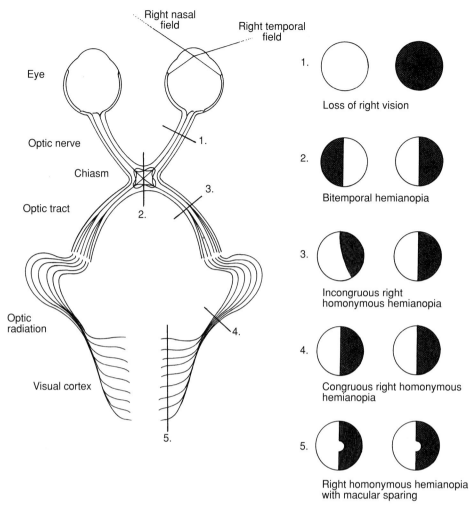

Fig. 153
Field of vision defects in relation to the anatomical pathway.

form the efferent part of the reflex that runs in the third nerve to constrict the pupil (Fig. 154). Adie's and third nerve palsies are defects of the efferent or outflow aspect of the pupil reflex. The pupil is innervated by sympathetic (dilation) and parasympathetic stimuli (constriction). Horner's syndrome is an anomaly of the sympathetic innervation of the pupil.

Horner's syndrome

If the sympathetic nerve supply to the face is damaged, the patient develops Horner's syndrome (Fig. 155). This can be caused by:

- neck trauma
- Pancoast's tumour (apical lung carcinoma)
- congenital defect
- idiopathic defect (probably vascular).

Clinical features
The characteristic features of Horner's syndrome are a small pupil, slight ptosis and reduced sweating of the skin on the ipsilateral side of the face.

Diagnosis
Chest X-ray and possible bronchoscopy are indicated.

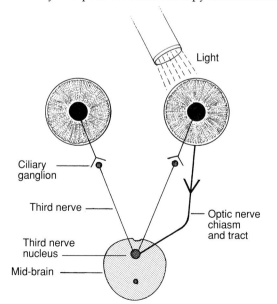

Fig. 154
The pupillary light pathway.

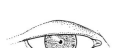
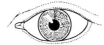

Fig. 155
Right Horner's syndrome.

Management
No specific treatment is possible.

Adie's pupil

In Adie's pupil, the affected pupil is dilated. This usually affects young women. A viral infection of the ciliary ganglion is the probable cause.

Clinical features
The affected pupil is dilated and does not react (either directly or consensually) to light. It does react slowly to accommodation and tends to remain miosed for a prolonged period after accommodating.

The eye movements are full.

Management
This is a benign condition and reassurance is essential. Although the accommodative response is present, it is commonly reduced and the patient may require assistance, with glasses for reading.

Complications
The other eye commonly becomes affected.

Third nerve palsy

The pupil is dilated and does not react to light or accommodation either directly or consensually (see under strabismus).

Afferent defect

If there is an anomaly of the afferent limb of the pupil response, i.e. macula or optic nerve, then the consensual pupillary response on the affected side is stronger than the direct response (Fig. 156).

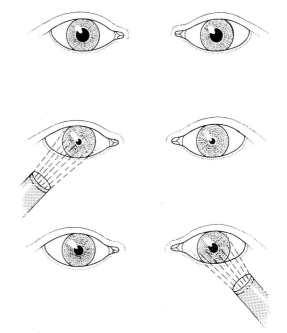

Fig. 156
An afferent pupillary defect. The consensual response of the left pupil is stronger than the direct response.

Clinical features
The vision is usually poor in the affected eye. The direct response to light is diminished. This may be obvious, but more subtle defects can be picked up by swinging the light stimulus briskly to and fro between each eye and watching for any change in the response. The affected pupil will appear to dilate when the light is shone directly into it as the direct response is much weaker (Fig. 156).

Diagnosis
Fundal examination for retinal or optic nerve disease and optic nerve imaging may be necessary.

Management
Management depends on the cause of the problem.

Self-assessment: questions

Multiple choice questions

1. Optic atrophy may be caused by:
   a. Blunt ocular trauma
   b. Optic neuritis
   c. Ischaemic optic neuropathy
   d. Glaucoma
   e. An occipital lobe infarct

2. Compression of the optic chiasm:
   a. Usually causes a homonymous hemianopia
   b. May be associated with acromegaly
   c. May present with a headache
   d. Is common in Down's syndrome
   e. Causes a squint

3. The following field of vision defects and pathological entities are commonly associated with one another:
   a. Loss of central vision in the right eye and Horner's syndrome
   b. Left homonymous hemianopia with an intracranial tumour
   c. Loss of inferior field in the right eye with a pituitary tumour
   d. Loss of superior field in the left eye with giant cell arteritis
   e. Bitemporal hemianopia and cerebrovascular accidents

4. Anisocoria (unequal pupils) may be caused by:
   a. Sixth nerve palsy
   b. Horner's syndrome
   c. Adie's syndrome
   d. Pituitary adenomas
   e. Third nerve palsies

Case history

A 78-year-old man presents complaining that he cannot see out of his right eye. Visual acuities are 6/9 in each eye. He is known to have hypertension.

1. What may be the explanation for his symptoms?
2. How would you proceed with the examination?

Short notes

Write short notes on:

1. anterior ischaemic optic neuropathy
2. papilloedema
3. Horner's syndrome

Viva questions

1. What is optic neuritis?
2. Give two causes of optic neuritis
3. Give three causes of optic atrophy
4. Describe and draw the field defect in (a) a chiasmal lesion and (b) an occipital lesion.

Self-assessment: answers

Multiple choice questions

1. a. **True.** Severe blunt trauma may damage the blood supply to the optic nerve and result in optic atrophy.
   b. **True.** Optic neuritis is a common cause of optic atrophy.
   c. **True.** Ischaemic optic neuropathy is a common cause of optic atrophy.
   d. **True.** Glaucoma causes cupping and atrophy of the optic nerve, which result in reduced vision.
   e. **False.** An infarct of the occipital lobe will not affect the optic nerve, but will result in a homonymous hemianopia.

2. a. **False.** Lesions of the optic chiasm characteristically cause a bitemporal hemianopia.
   b. **True.**
   c. **True.** Presentation is usually because of headache, hormonal disturbance (e.g. acromegaly) or awareness of visual loss.
   d. **False.** There is no association with Down's syndrome.
   e. **False.** Squints are not caused by the lesion.

3. a. **False.** Horner's syndrome has no effect on the field of vision: it is an interruption of the sympathetic supply to the eye.
   b. **True.** Other causes are infarction and infection.
   c. **False.**
   d. **True.** Altitudinal defects which may affect the upper or lower field of vision in one eye are usually vascular in aetiology—one of the causes being giant cell arteritis.
   e. **False.** Pituitary tumours classically cause bitemporal hemianopias due to pressure on the optic chiasm; the blood supply to the chiasm is excellent, therefore cerebrovascular accidents are not a cause of damage to the area.

4. a. **False.** The sixth nerve does not innervate the pupil.
   b. **True.** This affects the sympathetic nerve supply to the eye and causes a miosed pupil on the affected side.
   c. **True.** This causes interruption of the parasympathetic innervation of the eye and therefore causes a larger pupil on the affected side.
   d. **False.**
   e. **True.**

Case history answer

1. The most likely explanation for this gentlemen's problem is a right-sided homonymous hemianopia. This is probably due to a small cerebrovascular accident secondary to hypertension. Patients often mistake a homonymous hemianopia for loss of vision in the eye of the affected side.
2. Testing the fields of vision to confrontation should confirm the clinical diagnosis.

Short notes answers

1. Anterior ischaemic optic neuropathy is a condition that predominantly affects the elderly population. The presentation is of sudden painless reduction in vision affecting one eye. The optic nerve head appears swollen and there are haemorrhages around the posterior pole of the eye. The condition may be caused by arteritis or atherosclerosis. It is vital to determine which type the patient has, as the arteritic variety should be treated immediately with high doses of systemic steroids to prevent the other eye becoming affected. Therefore, the plasma viscosity or ESR must be measured as an emergency in such patients. The prognosis for visual recovery is poor.
2. Papilloedema is swelling of the optic nerve head caused by raised intracranial pressure. The patient often has no ocular symptoms but usually presents with headache. On examination, the optic disc is elevated and there are haemorrhages around the margins of the disc. The patient requires intracranial imaging (CT or MRI).
3. Horner's syndrome is a triad of a unilateral small pupil, ptosis and reduced sweating on that side of the face. It is caused by an interruption of the sympathetic nerve supply to that side of the face. The most common cause is idiopathic, presumed vascular, but lung cancer and neck trauma may also cause the syndrome.

Viva answers

1. This is an inflammation of the optic nerve that causes a progressive reduction in vision, associated with pain on moving the eye. Visual recovery, which takes place over a period of 1–4 weeks, is the normal course of the disease.
2. Any two of: demyelination, viral infection or idiopathic causes.
3. Optic atrophy may be secondary to: optic nerve tumours, optic neuritis, ischaemic optic neuropathy, chronic papilloedema, optic nerve trauma or ocular disease that damages the optic nerve head.
4. The field defect in chiasmal compression is termed a bitemporal hemianopia and the field defect in an occipital lesion is termed a homonymous hemianopia (see Fig. 153 for drawings).

Index